T0208911

# WHO CAN PARENTS TRUST?

Vaccines: Avoidable and Unsafe

David Denton Davis, MD

BALBOA.
PRESS

A DIVISION OF HAY HOUSE

Balboa Press books may be ordered through booksellers or by contacting:

Balboa Press
A Division of Hay House
1663 Liberty Drive
Bloomington, IN 47403
www.balboapress.com
1 (877) 407-4847

Print information available on the last page.

ISBN: 978-1-9822-0439-6 (sc)
ISBN: 978-1-9822-0437-2 (hc)
ISBN: 978-1-9822-0438-9 (e)

Library of Congress Control Number: 2018905806

Balboa Press rev. date: 06/18/2018

# Contents

# Introduction

## Who can parents trust?

My intention in writing this book is plain and simple. I am asking for everyone to understand we are dealing with a pandemic of unimaginable proportions that is having a devastating effect on our children and grandchildren. Diseases seldom before seen are now rampant with no meaningful explanations coming from our medical profession. While our leading experts appear to be in total denial about what has been allowed to happen in the name of eradicating childhood illnesses, a worldwide non-infectious growing toxic plague has descended upon both our young and old. The seeds were planted with the introduction of pesticides without concern about the impact on nature or humanity. A bestselling author, Rachel Carson, took on the petrochemical giant Monsanto by writing an incredibly detailed story documenting the danger of DDT and its impact on our food chain. Publishers initially turned their backs on *The Silent Spring* due to fear. Carson's message was clear what we were doing to nature we were doing to ourselves because everything in nature is interconnected. Although Monsanto mocked her work, President John F. Kennedy stood by her inescapable evidence and further use of DDT was soon banned in America.

Today, I believe we are dealing with a far more dangerous situation in regard to vaccines. Carson was concerned about tampering with nature, but I am now more concerned about direct tampering with human beings. Those diseases not previously known have risen in parallel with the introduction and escalation in the administration of vaccines combined with an unprecedented first year of life vaccine schedule. I realize there will be profound implications inherent in asking for an immediate halt to our current vaccine program, but I do not believe we have any other choice. The facts do not lie. Key ingredients being injected into mothers-to-be, newborns, infants and children typically found in vaccines, especially aluminum and mercury, have never been proven safe for humans. Studies I have looked at carefully that have been conducted to prove there are no serious vaccine adverse side effects have, in my humble medical opinion, failed. Frankly speaking the results are frightening and cannot be ignored. I had hoped another President would have the courage to live up to a promise. That is not about to happen due to money and inevitable liability. No one in power can afford to see the obvious or speak out if they have.

Stopping this pandemic that has been created by our pharmaceutical industry with help from petrochemical giants like Monsanto will not be easy without a full blown product boycott by humanity in the name of sanity. Every day I hear and see more concerned parents, doctors, nurses, scientists and lawyers speaking out about informed consent, First Amendment and civil rights. Implementing and standing by these rights must be our first step.

Who can parents trust? The final chapter and paragraph in my 2010 book, *Dancing Cats Silent Canaries* ended with this question. Based upon research, I had concluded no governmental agency or medical organization could afford to admit any responsibility for our currently growing neurological, gastrointestinal, cardiovascular and immunological epidemics affecting all ages. There are explanations. More likely than not, causes are rooted in known environmental toxins, certain vaccines, vaccine combinations, their adjuvants and our immunization schedule doctors and parents are being told to follow. Prior to and since writing that book, I have wanted to believe new evidence would emerge vaccines are safe. I cannot say there has and remain truthful. Looking closely at vaccine created serious adverse events combined with widespread outbreaks of childhood illnesses among those vaccinated provides us with sufficient evidence artificially induced immunity using adjuvants considered poisons can be neither safe nor effective. Parents cannot trust doctors who claim vaccines are safe and effective for all. Doctors can no longer afford to trust medical experts, who profess deaths and illnesses following vaccinations, are purely coincidental. Medical experts, health agencies and doctors financially benefiting from vaccines have a conflict of interest making these people and entities totally untrustworthy.

What follows is about truth, trust, coincidence, consequence, correlations and cause. Neither doctors nor parents have been told the whole truth about possible harm that can befall an infant, child, or adult following administration of either single or multiple vaccines. Multiple vaccines, especially those containing aluminum, are far more dangerous than single vaccines. Research is readily available on the subject of known neurotoxic properties of aluminum and mercury. Naturally acquired immunity from exposure and illness becomes lasting. Once an illness has passed our immune systems have a chance to be bolstered by future exposures. Artificial immunity, which depends on adjuvants and an array of other unnecessary ingredients, has precipitated epidemics of disease and death. Unfortunately, rather than attribute an adverse event to consequence following vaccination, coincidence is, more often than not, used.

Before going into more ominous detail, I would like to apologize to parents who have an infant or child who has sustained a deadly or disabling probable vaccine related injury. As an Emergency physician, I could have done so much more to raise concerns about vaccine awareness, if I had only known more about timing and toxic ingredients. Timing is about any death or illness that occurs within hours, days or weeks of a vaccine or vaccine combination. By law I should have identified a date when vaccine injections were last given and made out a report if it had been within thirty days of an emergency visit. My responsibility was to report possible adverse events not to blame any vaccinations. I failed to do so. If I was aware toxins, including mercury and aluminum, were being injected into babies in increasing amounts, in accordance with a growing vaccine schedule, I probably would not have allowed my children to be injected. Fortunately, forty years ago they received ninety-nine percent less total mercury and aluminum by age two than today.

In spite of the fact vaccine package inserts list problems, previously reported as adverse events, likely caused by vaccines or vaccine ingredients, our medical community has been paying little or no attention to this available information. Any physician, physician assistant, nurse practitioner, nurse or pharmacist, who continues to believe manufacturer acknowledged adverse events are just coincidences, cannot be trusted. Any media reports suggesting vaccines are safe and effective should be ignored. Doctors who have come to their own conclusions suggesting vaccines, combinations, adjuvants, ingredients and schedule are not safe for all should be heard.

With growing evidence of vaccine harm available ten years ago, I proposed it was time to invoke the *Precautionary Principle*. Shifting proof for vaccine product safety to an industry already immune from liability was not about to happen. Notwithstanding manufacturer warnings to the contrary, childhood vaccines were considered one of our greatest medical accomplishments of the Twentieth Century. No one wanted to believe there was a darker more sinister side, likely associated with vaccine ingredients that were contributing to a surge in infant deaths, neurological disabilities and a growing list of autoimmune illnesses. Knowing I was very naïve believing the *Precautionary Principle* might be invoked allowing for additional proofs for safety, my attention turned to the vaccine safety net, known as our Vaccine Adverse Event Reporting System (VAERS). Reasonably concluding serious vaccine induced adverse events would, more likely than not, show up in emergency departments, I shifted my attention. Without exposing a real number for serious adverse events nothing would ever change. Emergency department based VAERS counts taking place over twelve consecutive months would likely show the seriousness of our vaccine problem. Another possibility was it would not make any difference, simply because doctors and parents favoring vaccine safety really don't want to know about a serious downside.

Before and after my first book, I attempted to obtain adverse event reporting help from emergency physicians. I quickly learned very few knew anything about vaccine related adverse events or our reporting procedure. As a result, I had every reason to conclude things might be much different today, if medicine's gatekeepers, as we liked to call ourselves in the early days, had received information about our reporting responsibilities. If we had been included in 1986, we may have forced invocation of the *Precautionary Principle* long ago. In essence, I believed a mandatory reporting component, which helped offer vaccine manufacturer freedom from product liability, would have quickly provided proof vaccine harm was vastly exceeding hoped for benefits.

At the time I had been prompted to look more closely at adverse events, when my youngest daughter asked me if I knew of any reason four horses had suddenly died without explanation. Her hunch was each animal had received multiple vaccines before leaving a horse show. Each died suddenly in trailers hauling them home. I knew she was probably correct. Four horses just don't succumb and die hours after injections for no identifiable reason. Then my youngest son, on my advice, said no thank you to a hep B on the day Andrew was born. Neither the nursery nurse nor Andrew's pediatrician gracefully accepted his informed decision. Initial disdain was followed with disrespect on the occasion of my grandson's well baby visit. His pediatrician, who had managed my granddaughter's lead toxicity by doing nothing, handed my son Andrew's medical records and advised him to go elsewhere. Somewhat shocked by his attitude my son backed down and submitted to prerequisite conditions. I understood and respected his decision. I had heard similar stories from many other mothers and fathers willing to relinquish control of their infants and children to their trusted pediatricians. I did not know pediatricians were being paid for their vaccine performance.

Although correlation does not equal causation the following chapters may shed new light on what I consider a shocking picture of a situation we as physicians and parents have allowed to get out of control. Physicians should have known better. Parents and caregivers cannot trust in doctors who insist all vaccines are safe for every child. Proponents are, for the most part, well meaning if they have not been touched by vaccine money. Unfortunately very few pediatricians can practice without income from their sale of vaccines. Ultimately, answers to our most profound questions on how serious our vaccine problem is may already have an answer. Going forward having emergency physicians trigger VAERS submissions would be one way to show what has been happening. However, there may be a far simpler way to have truth about vaccine damage consequences revealed in a shorter period;

namely, a retrospective analysis. I believe evidence can be found today within medical records and insurance claim forms of babies dying or becoming seriously ill in those hours, days and weeks following their vaccinations. Readers will soon learn about our VAERS database which already contains reported information about infant deaths within days or weeks of a vaccine. Reports generated by third party administrators, a component of our insurance industry, have provided a glimpse at what I see may be an answer to our vaccine problem's magnitude.

Insurance companies known to financially reward doctors and hospitals for keeping patients up to date in accordance with vaccine schedule demand may in truth be hiding incriminating evidence. This means insurance companies, including those federally funded to provide coverage for both our indigent and elderly already have what needs to be known in their databases. Therefore, I am positive evidence of vaccine harm for many infants, children and adults is available and accessible in their files. Can anyone believe our insurance industry would deliberately withhold crucial information pertaining to their beneficiaries overall health?

Analysis of only a very small sample may reveal the true size of what I consider a vaccine injury iceberg. Choosing Mississippi Medicaid recipients medical records for a vaccine audit, I believe, will show overwhelming evidence of illnesses and deaths following vaccinations. I am certain the reasons why this state has America's unhealthiest children and highest infant death rate will be found. Data will not prove with certainty vaccines were responsible, but it will show how many serious adverse events were never reported to VAERS. Simply extrapolating Mississippi's data to forty nine states will reveal what lies below the surface and will expose vaccine safety is a myth.

Another source for vaccine safety information might come from the Pediatrix Group. Pediatrix provides Neonatal Intensive Care Unit (NICU) services for more than 400 hospitals in all fifty states. Readers will soon learn about a five year retrospective study on the process and results for bringing 14,000 extremely low birth weight (ELBW) infants up to date on their required two month of age vaccinations using multiple same day injections. Many serious adverse events were documented over a five year period. In spite of their findings no reason was found to recommend any changes in vaccine types, numbers or schedule. We should be able to conclude Pediatrix physicians knew all about VAERS, so many answers will likely be found in their database, if these serious vaccines related events were documented, but never reported. Identifying what happened to these premature infants in years following their injections and discharge would be of extraordinary value, especially if they all remained healthy. Unfortunately, for these infants evidence has come to light adult men getting similar multiple vaccines are showing signs of physical cellular damage.

In chapters following my intention is to build an ethical and moral case favoring reasons why parents must not trust anyone but themselves. Hopefully, my story will be of help for parents, caregivers and healthcare professionals being confronted by mandates and threats, to rely instead on their right to self determination. Both our First Amendment and Civil Rights legislation guarantee personal and religious freedom of choice. Mississippi, West Virginia and California have legislatively chosen to abolish these rights in the name of vaccines. When evidence suggests adverse events associated with submitting to vaccines or a schedule represent individual risks greater than collective benefits, everyone deserves being heard. Refusing a vaccine based upon informed consent must remain an individual's protected right. Medical exemptions, submitted on behalf of infants and parents, by concerned physicians, will increasingly become necessary and critically important to assure personal safety and to avoid suggestions of malfeasance for failing to do so. Vaccine control may be more important than gun control.

Parents and caregivers should never have been placed in this quandary, if physicians, health agencies, health insurance carriers, media and law makers had not chosen to abandon their trust, in return for monetary rewards from a vaccine industry now apparently above our laws. While protective parents and caregivers exercise their right to informed consent and possible need for medical exemptions for their children, I am hopeful more and more physicians will realize babies' lives matter more than vaccine makers or their own practice profit.

Doctors must become aware serious adverse events following exposure to vaccines and vaccine combinations represent a danger makers have already acknowledged can happen. No matter how rare is irrelevant. Existing databases will reveal these serious adverse events are far more common than ever imaginable. Of greater importance is to know more about longer term outcomes in these select groups. There is no honest scientific study proving increasing vaccine use does not correlate with our growing autism epidemic or our high infant death rate. State law makers attempting mandatory vaccination regulations must be stopped before every state becomes another Mississippi unless hidden insurance data becomes available proving vaccines are not responsible.

Parents must also consider other risk factor dangers posed by pesticides, such as Glyphosate and PVC plastic crib mattresses containing arsenic and antimony. Like our vaccine makers, our chemical manufacturers have no honest concern about anyone or anything other than their own selfish interests in profitability. While parents and infants suffer, doctors are being warned not to attempt interventions on behalf of their patient's safety. I am hopeful this book will help more doctors come to the realization they have not been paying enough attention to what has been happening to medicine. At a time when petrochemical giants are pesticide poisoning our soil and fracking land beneath our feet and vaccine makers are doing the same to our children and our immune systems without liability, it is time for citizens to say no more.

Our tobacco industry's Master Settlement Agreement paid and continues to pay for damages caused by their products. Pesticide and vaccine makers without providing proof for safety must be made responsible for human damages being caused by their products. Highly paid industrial lobbyists and costly indemnification agreements cannot be allowed to continue to destroy our land and our children, respectively. Our 1986 National Childhood Vaccine Act (NCVIA) freeing makers from liability for injuries following use of their vaccine products must be repealed before it is too late for a third generation of children.

I would like to thank my wife Cynnea for her daily love and perseverance with me and my efforts to reveal what is being hidden in order to bring an end to the continued use of toxic vaccines. I am equally proud of her efforts on behalf of Autism Tree Project Foundation and Art and Autism. I remain thankful my younger brother, a victim of still to be banned asbestos induced Mesothelioma, for his continued inspiration from above.

# 1

## Evidence of Vaccine Harm Abounds

Once I learned there could be vaccine induced adverse events, I began to see everyday evidence. Adverse event expectations became part of my history taking for every child with a fever, nausea, vomiting, rash, lethargy, irritability or seizure. A correlation between illnesses and recent shots became immediately evident. At the very least my medical records now had additional information and a child's parents would know I was aware this might also be their concern. I was soon amazed at the numbers of illnesses which qualified as possible vaccine related adverse events.

A short time after my son's pediatric encounter, I entered an urgent care exam room where a young febrile boy experiencing uncontrollable face and neck movements was waiting. I asked his mother whether her son had received any recent vaccinations. Surprised by my question she replied, "Three days ago." Recognizing his uncontrollable tics were seizures, I questioned when they started. "In church on Sunday, two days after his MMR," was her reply. I immediately contacted their pediatrician. What followed was shocking. After I suggested her patient was suffering from an adverse event, she reprimanded me by saying it was not due to his vaccine. She added that her office did not do reports. I asked if she could tell me what VAERS actually meant. My phone went silent.

I was thrown back onto my prior journey in search of truth about what I had been witnessing, but apparently missing for more than twenty five years. Years earlier on a flight, I remembered talking with an anesthesiologist, who mentioned his fifteen year old son had Tourette's syndrome while we were talking about vaccine induced adverse events. He realized his son had experienced a sudden major exacerbation in tics following his DPT booster prior to summer camp. He asked if it was a coincidence, although he was now certain it was a likely DPT consequence without possibility of proving a correlation.

During subsequent years many more examples have occurred convincing me beyond any doubt causes for our current troubles have been subjected to a continuing cover-up in the name of society's greater good. Our best opportunity to alter course in the name of infant and childhood safety passed by when a group of our most intelligent leaders met and, perhaps, reluctantly agreed the consequences stemming from any admission vaccine products might be unsafe were far too great. There could be no continued legal protection from liability for our pharmaceutical industry, if so called peer reviewed scientific articles proving safety, were shown to be fraudulent.

Rather than deal with evidence and likely consequences vaccine makers were given a free pass. Over the next ten years an unfolding tragedy has continued with a further doubling in our nation's autism rate and no decline in unexplained infant deaths. In 2003 our prestigious Institute of Medicine (IOM) likely had contrary evidence, but chose to ignore it by silence. Any admission worldwide vaccine programs were, perhaps, causing more harm than good would have to wait. With a statement that the evidence favors rejection of a causal relationship between exposure to multiple vaccinations and sudden infant death syndrome (SIDS), our IOM hoped would put any lingering questions about vaccine safety to rest. Several known studies that suggested a temporal relationship existed between vaccines, SIDS and autism in a certain population subset would need to be ignored.

The United States remains number one in the world in infant deaths and first year vaccinations. This cannot be just a coincidence. Is it possible members of that select committee meeting in secrecy became frightened? Was it possible members were warned about legal risks associated with any admission a significant percentage of more than one million SIDS cases worldwide were possibly caused by vaccines? Or, is it plausible they actually knew vaccine dangers, but concluded there would be no immediate forthcoming proof for a mechanism of injury? After that meeting some members suggested there needed to be a study to determine existence of a more vaccine vulnerable subset of infants, although nothing would be done. Without admitting internal discussions favored a more definitive statement, IOM members agreed to silence.

Unsurprisingly many participants refused to sign their committee's conclusion to do nothing. It is unlikely they did not know there was a lack of science behind vaccine safety or our CDC's acclaimed Danish study showing no link between vaccines and autism was fraudulent. Nevertheless, they wanted everyone to believe no further safety studies needed to be done. Their titanic decision was full speed ahead, perhaps, suggesting a few babies' lives don't matter. Reasons favoring rejection may have been influenced by strong possibilities newer studies would add to already accumulating evidence of vaccine harm. Their recommendation that no further studies should be done was likely an admission there was fear about what would be found.

Meanwhile, where do we as parents, grandparents and physicians currently stand? Where can well meaning doctors go to learn the truth? When will doctors, who have conducted studies purporting there is no correlation between vaccine contents death and disability, come forward and acknowledge their conclusions may have been wrong, or performed for the wrong reasons. We already know where our leadership stands. It is more apparent than ever to understand parents can only trust themselves. Parents must become informed enough to resist being bullied by medical doctors or our media. Causality will eventually flow from a series of correlations.

Following an email link, I watched a video depicting a story of a healthy vibrant twenty month old boy who died a week after his tetanus, diphtheria and pertussis (TDaP) shot. His mother, a registered nurse, spoke out blaming the vaccine. She reported he was not himself in the days following, but seemed to be rallying only to be found face down cold cuddled up dead in his crib. I cried. I had previously been vilified by a pediatric pathologist for suggesting on network news there was nothing natural about unexplained infant deaths. I knew there had to be a correlation between SIDS, environmental toxins and especially vaccines and their ingredients.

Perhaps, I should have gone beyond the recommendations made to parents in 2010. Delaying all vaccinations until year two or beyond may have saved Nicholas. I was even more ashamed when I learned this twenty month old child's autopsy was likely no different than those performed thirty years ago. Studies requested by a nurse were simply ignored and death was attributed to natural causes. In spite of evidence death was not natural or a coincidence, a coroner made a clear statement it was not vaccine related. How can any death not be allowed to correlate with a temporal event such as a TDaP vaccination? The manufacturer already attests in their vaccine insert reports of some babies dying from SIDS following their TDaP vaccine. Should we ignore vaccine makers? Why would vaccine makers lie?

It is unlikely there were any measurements made of C-reactive protein (CRP) or cytokine levels, such as interleukin 6 (IL6) in Nicholas' body at the time of death. Scientific studies going back to 1996 have shown strikingly high levels of these inflammatory markers, especially in boys, post-vaccination, including TDaP injections. CRP and IL6 are typically high in association with brain inflammation; namely, encephalitis. Manufacturers have warned us about a possible occurrence of this serious adverse event (AE). Doesn't anyone care to listen to or believe when manufacturers tell us encephalitis can be a post-vaccination possibility which can go on to become disabling or deadly? When a manufacturer lists sudden infant death and autism as reported pre-marketing adverse events, everyone needs to heed the warning. Here are several paragraphs from the TDaP (Tripedia) vaccine package insert;

"In the German case-control study and US open-label safety study in which 14,971 infants received Tripedia vaccine, 13 deaths in Tripedia vaccine recipients were reported. Causes of deaths included seven SIDS one cardiac arrest....."

"Adverse events reported during post-approval use of Tripedia vaccine include idiopathic thrombocytopenic purpura, SIDS, anaphylactic reaction, cellulitis, autism, convulsion/grand mal convulsion, encephalopathy, hypotonia, neuropathy, somnolence and apnea. Events were included in this list because of the seriousness….."

Additional adverse reactions:

"As with other aluminum-containing vaccines, a nodule may be palpable at the injection sites for several weeks. Sterile abscess formation at the site of injection has been reported. Rarely, an anaphylactic reaction, hives, swelling of the mouth, difficulty breathing, hypotension, or shock has been reported after receiving preparations containing diphtheria, tetanus, and/or pertussis antigens.

Words attempting to minimize these revelations were used; however, I believe the thing speaks for itself. When a manufacturer uses SIDS and autism as possible serious adverse events everyone, especially doctors, need to pay closer attention. I do not believe any parent or caregiver would consent to the risk of SIDS, if they read or were informed of this risk by a healthcare worker. The real question might be if autism today affects one in every thirty-six live births, how many have been termed a TDaP vaccine consequence? Those of us practicing in emergency departments may have been able to make this real time correlation, if we had asked the right questions and received correct answers. It is never too late to look back and take some positive long overdue action. Unless we as physicians choose to listen to vaccine maker warnings and parent suspicions, ultimately we may be construed as accomplices.

During 2016 in America there were 6.1 first year infant deaths for every 1,000 live births. Sudden unexplained infant death (SUID) and sudden unexplained childhood deaths (SUCD) are more than likely in a majority of cases explainable with the word vaccines. Once there was only SIDS. After infant deaths in the 1950's began to mount without any specific identifiable clinical findings revealing a cause these words were created in order to justify a diagnostic code. Babies dying after age two months and before age twelve months without an autopsy identifiable cause were diagnosed as SIDS.

When a similar lack of a cause for deaths began to occur in infants older than twelve months twenty years ago this new SUCD diagnosis appeared. SIDS became a SUID subgroup. A SIDS diagnosis was used when no cause was identified for death after autopsy, death scene investigation and review of the family history. Infants were categorized as SUID before any thorough investigation. SUID also includes cases of infant deaths from unknown cause. This group might include those not investigated completely or cases of suffocation or strangulation in bed. In 2015 there were 3,700 SUIDs of which 1,600 were determined to be SIDS and 1,200 as cause unknown, leaving about 900 in the strangulation category. In other words more than three out of four deaths were not explainable. Zero deaths were attributed to vaccines. How is it possible, when TDaP makers acknowledge reports of SIDS, physicians are not able to find one case? Parents or daycare workers without evidence have been found guilty of killing infants, while vaccines with probable evidence of harm are consistently found innocent.

What constitutes a suspected SIDS exam? Without tissue, blood, and spinal fluid examination for mercury, lead, arsenic, antimony, aluminum, inflammatory markers, other toxins and perhaps, cholinesterase activity, a post mortem is, in my medical opinion, incomplete. Any death scene investigation that fails to examine anything found in a child's crib, including the mattress, is at best inconclusive. Without going into detail there is a possibility an infant with a vaccine induced febrile illness sleeping on an older crib mattress may be in greatest danger. An interaction between mold contaminated PVC mattresses may adversely affect a sleeping infant's cardio-respiratory function. This interaction has been scientifically studied for more than one hundred and fifty years.

Statistically eliminating victims older than twelve months made it seem our incidence of SIDS was declining when in fact actual numbers were increasing. Incomplete investigations also allowed for reclassification into the SUID group. Babies dying for no apparent reason before age two months, if completely investigated, would increase SIDS numbers. Evidence now suggests deaths before age two months may be attributable to the introduction of a day of birth hep B vaccine. For unknown reasons, statistical correlations between SIDS and vaccines have largely been ignored. Why does Japan have only two infant deaths per 1,000 live births? Is it due to fewer vaccines? Why do thirty two other countries have fewer than six infant deaths per 1,000 live births? Do these countries give fewer vaccines? Yes is a correct answer for either of these questions. How many of our infant deaths received a vaccine hours, days or weeks preceding death? I am convinced insurance companies have an answer to this question. I want to know how many actually died within thirty days of receiving any vaccine or vaccine combination.

Sadly, the numbers of sickened babies not dying for medically explainable reasons has been simultaneously growing into explainable epidemics. Mechanisms causing death in some and disability in many may be similar; namely, too many vaccines, too much aluminum and too many toxins being given much too soon. A study in Mississippi, where vaccine compliance is at 99.4%, shows our country's highest incidence of unhealthy children with an infant death rate 25% higher than our national average. A well known doctor and vaccine inventor, Paul Offit, admitted these numbers are puzzling. If he would like a reasonable explanation he might join a movement that will ask for this state's help. Answers will likely be found using a data sample from Medicaid.

After reading several depressing peer reviewed studies, I felt my time had come to write a new book correlating details and piecing together facts in order to help parents, caregivers and doctors better understand what I see. I believe enough evidence is in plain sight. Evidence suggests vaccines are lethal for some but obviously not all. A need to halt or slow vaccine administrations will be based upon peer reviewed extremely low birth weight baby studies, which I believe cannot be ignored or dismissed. A painstaking review of several existing scientific studies may offer both parents and doctors help in deciding reasons for concern beyond Mississippi. I believe there is evidence available proving a correlation exists between mandated vaccines and adverse event study results. Evidence vaccines are a root cause of harm statistically abounds in correlating vaccination dates in these studies and those found in medical records and insurance claim forms.

# 2

Have We Gotten
Out of Control?

There appears to be pre-occupation complying with a vaccine schedule which makes little or no sense. Making hep B vaccine, for example, a first day of life event to prevent a blood borne disease found mainly in drug users, prostitutes and our gay community is so ridiculous it needs no comment. For physicians or nurses to give hep B to premature babies confined in NICU's borders on obsessive compulsive behavior. Notwithstanding existing peer reviewed warnings, this vaccine is being routinely given every day even in countries with no known hepatitis B risks.

A retrospective study published in 2015 actually documented serious adverse events following vaccinations given to extremely low birth weight (ELBW) infants. This study covered a five year period. The traditional medical belief, when it comes to vaccines that infant birth weight, gestational age and genetic framework make no difference, based upon reported results, is fundamentally wrong. Any study which documents serious life threatening consequences following vaccine administration cannot be disregarded, especially when a study's stated purpose is there would be none. It is also important to emphasize same day serious vaccine adverse events reported in ELBW babies can have similar affects on normal birth weight infants. The only difference, in my medical opinion, is infants who go home following their initial hep

B shot or their scheduled two month injections are not being monitored for changes in breathing, heart rate or oxygen levels. Except during sleep caregivers are the only effective monitors. Slowing heart rates, respirations and falling oxygen levels during sleep can lead to sudden death in all age groups.

This adverse event vaccine study published in a well known medical journal shows our medical establishment's ruthless denial that vaccines can and do cause harm. When I read the details, I was appalled. Again, in my opinion, this study is an example of vaccine medicine totally out of control. As marvelous as a human body is survival and continued function depends on normally functioning immune and detoxification systems. Ingredients in vaccines, especially aluminum, can confuse our immune system, overwhelm detoxification pathways and injure developing brains resulting in death or immune and neurological injury. Data clearly shows male infants are most vulnerable, perhaps accounting for predictable higher incidences of SIDS and autism.

Anyone who dares argue an extremely low birth weight (ELBW) infant has fully functioning immune, kidney and detoxification abilities does not have a basic understanding of either an infant's immune system or biochemistry pathways. For that matter, anyone who believes a normally appearing one year old child has successfully developed these same capabilities is also wrong. Therefore, perhaps no child under age three has an ability to successfully defend against or excrete any potentially toxic ingredients typically found in vaccines, not to mention their own crib environments.

It might be fair to conclude members attending that 2003 Simpsonwood secret IOM meeting did not know either vaccine manufacturers' warnings or emerging NICU studies showing unexpected outcomes. Or, perhaps they did. Studies focused upon babies hospitalized due to premature births deserve special consideration. Researchers' conclusions may be of greater concern. Oftentimes, doctors read study summaries in an abstract or go directly to authors' conclusions about their findings with no attention given to graphic presentations or a study's process. Common sense may reveal all conclusions cannot be justified by either process or results.

Most studies are done under Institutional Review Board (IRB) approval. An IRB can be located within or outside a healthcare facility. Approval is usually predicated upon risks and potential benefits. Study quality can be considered excellent, if outcomes confirm the author's original expectations, without causing harm. Obviously, any scientific study can have a serious downside, if there are unexpected adverse consequences or unexplained clinical findings during the process. For example, I was a member of a pharmaceutical research group retained by a drug company with IRB approval to give an intravenous drug to a certain group of stoke victims. Obtaining signed patient or family approval without giving any guarantee a product would be beneficial prior to administration was essential. If study data suggested our product seemed to benefit outcomes without doing any harm conclusions would become self evident. In this particular study a benefit was not statistically proven.

During another major 1990's academic study the authors' speculated a new heart medication given immediately following a heart attack would lessen the risk for cardiac arrest. No one knew which patients would receive drug or placebo. Unfortunately, it became apparent within a short period heart attack victims receiving the drug were dying more frequently than those getting a placebo. This Boston based study was appropriately shut down simply because it was unethical and too dangerous to continue. In other words, an outcome was unexpected that showed this drug was harmful. Death became a consequence rather than a coincidence.

In one last IRB example a Harvard affiliated pediatric colleague proposed a study that involved children with Thalassemia major (TM), a rare inevitably fatal genetic disease. Children born with this disease destroy their own and any transfused red blood cells releasing in the process iron. Iron accumulates in body organs, including the skin, invariably resulting in organ failure deaths before age ten. This genetic disease is 100% fatal.

Nonetheless, a pediatric physician with help from private investors came up with an automated intravenous infusion pump designed to constantly administer a drug that would capture iron and escort it out of body organs through detoxification, kidney and gastrointestinal pathways. Without changing a fatal genetic disease, iron was effectively removed from victim's bodies with dramatic skin color changes and improved organ function. A study without apparent risk was shown to indefinitely prolong life.

This IRB approved study was closely scrutinized by other academic physicians. The author's conclusion lives were being saved was challenged, perhaps, due to the fact he was using a treatment called chelating therapy. It seems chelating therapy had been rendered an alternative medical term frowned upon by traditional doctors. Some medical experts suggested improvements in quality of life for these children were coincidental. Although TM victims were surviving, there was no absolute proof iron chelation was the reason. As preposterous as this may seem, there were physicians unable to accept this pediatrician's results, published in the New England Journal of Medicine (NEJM), were truly scientific. More will be said about fixed viewpoints, IRBs and approved vaccine experiments on ELBW infants. Parents and Thallasemia victims, whose lives were indefinitely prolonged, were thankful. One Saudi chelation patient later became a father whose son did not have this dominant genetic disease. Parental trust in this case was earned by a pediatrician choosing to defy traditional thinking by stepping out of medicine's proverbial box. The pump used became hematology's invention of the year.

Whenever risks appear to out weight benefit, I believe IRB's are morally and ethically obligated to intervene and bring any study to a halt. If a retrospective study not requiring IRB approval reveals significant harm may have occurred to some infants, there is no justification to repeat similar studies using an IRB. There is every reason to determine long term infant outcomes for an illness or injury that became apparent during a study. For some reason vaccine studies have become an exception to this general rule.

# 3

---

# More IRB Approved
# NICU Studies

Since choosing to publish my observations about our epidemics of sudden infant death, neurological and autoimmune diseases, I have witnessed a continued escalation. I have watched greater good propaganda bombardment at a time fully vaccinated children and young adults are experiencing a resurrection of childhood illnesses, such as measles, mumps, whooping cough and chickenpox. I have listened to prominent traditional doctors, government officials and our mainstream media point to unvaccinated as the cause and encourage parents to rush in for another round of the same apparently ineffective shots. How stupid do they think we are? I also see stories emerging from doctors our medical establishment label as non-traditional. A growing number are board certified pediatricians who are talking about their more healthy unvaccinated patients. I trust their observations are more honest than those pediatricians who cannot or else refuse to see their own evidence.

In my daily physician practice I see the havoc my profession has allowed to be wreaked upon more than two generations of children and adults. Daily I read posts written by mothers of children harmed by vaccines and concerned coalitions trying to warn us about what our government is doing to take away our First Amendment rights. I also read what pro-vaccine individuals have to say. Rather than defend vaccines they attack resistors. And then one morning I am sickened by reading a scientific peer reviewed vaccine study conducted by researchers with Duke University Medical Center's IRB approval. Before trying to explain objectives and conclusions of this study, I choose to point out a key pediatric researcher had ties and had previously received money from several pharmaceutical companies, including Glaxo Smith Kline (GSK).

Perhaps I should stop with the title *Adverse Events after Routine Immunization of Extremely Low-Birth-Weight Infants.* I should also provide a warning to readers about the content not being suitable for all. This study included 13,926 extremely low birth weight (ELBW) infants born at twenty eight weeks or less gestation, most of whom were discharged from January 1, 2007 to December 31, 2012. Ninety one percent of these infants received three vaccines. The incidence of sepsis in those receiving multiple vaccines increased four-fold in the days following. This means four times as many infants required invasive blood tests, antibiotics and much more to determine whether or not there were bacterial infections rather than vaccines causing the fevers. Infant rates for assisted breathing more than doubled in the hours following injection(s). This means assisting infants to breathe using masks with either room air or 100% oxygen. The numbers of infants requiring a tube to be placed in their windpipes (intubation) also doubled within three days of vaccinations which suggests their breathing became labored or stopped entirely (apnea). Slowing of infant heart rates (bradycardia) increased almost two-fold. Infants born at twenty three to twenty four weeks were reported by researchers to be at greater risk for these serious vaccine adverse events.

There is every reason to believe these same serious adverse events can be precursors of sudden infant deaths inside or outside a NICU. Study authors noted five infants died after receiving multiple immunizations. Their retrospective conclusion was these infants would have died anyway due to other medical causes. They went on to report one infant had a bowel perforation, another necrotizing intestinal disease and a third pneumonia. A cause of death for the final two was not reported for unexplained reasons. Five deaths were considered coincidental rather than a consequence of their vaccines.

I have a serious problem trying to understand how five very sick terminally ill infants were considered well enough by highly trained pediatricians to get their injections. I am also troubled by how any post- vaccination fatal illnesses could not be considered serious adverse consequences. What about the other two deaths, or does it matter? Perhaps, they died from sudden infant deaths.

In summary 13,926 hospitalized infants weighing less than 1000 grams (2.2 pounds) at birth participated in this retrospective analysis involving NICU's managed by the Pediatrix group during a five year period. In spite of their findings, study authors were able to conclude there was no valid reason not to give three or more vaccines at once. They reported there was a need for more studies to identify reasons for the unexpected numbers of vaccine related adverse events. Perhaps, instead of vaccines they should have been thinking about an IRB approved study limited only to aluminum injections for ELBW babies.

Researchers actually concluded the number and types of vaccines routinely given at two months of age, no matter how preposterous it may seem, should be considered safe. Although vaccinating ELBW infants in order to get them caught up with our recommended vaccine schedule is considered safe and necessary by our CDC, Advisory Committee on Immunization Practices (ACIP) and American Academy of Pediatrics (AAP), this study is frightening and reeks of the exact opposite. Perhaps, these researchers were so anxious to attach their names to a publication they didn't realize they had confirmed a problem already known to vaccine manufacturers and a growing list of parents.

Study authors stated there was no need to have informed consent for their study because it was retrospective. In other words data used was obtained from existing completed electronic medical records (EMR). Although these authors acknowledged prior smaller sample studies had shown ELBW infants had a significantly greater risk for vaccine adverse events than full term infants, they still did not see any problem with their results. They went on to conclude it would not be appropriate to make any changes in current practice. Although this study primarily analyzed data, it raises very serious and challenging questions when it comes to obtaining informed consent.

The first question might be were parents and caregivers for these babies ever informed about known increased vaccine risks before their babies were injected? It is unlikely 100%, after being told of a myriad of possible adverse events, all would have agreed. Next, were parents of those babies, who experienced serious consequences, advised that lifesaving measures became necessary? Thirdly, were any parents, whose babies suffered an adverse event, advised there might be a greater adverse event risk with their next vaccine? Were any parents told, as a result of the adverse events experienced by their premature babies, there might possibly be long term consequences?

One might ask researchers at Pediatrix, how their colleagues handled the parents of five dead babies? Were parents told vaccines were given before their babies died? Or were they told NICU pediatricians did not know how sick their babies were before giving them multiple shots? Were VAERS submissions completed for all babies who experienced a serious adverse event or for any of these five deaths? The authors acknowledged pneumococcal conjugate and TDaP vaccines were associated with more adverse events. Rather than admit their analysis confirmed prior scientific studies done in 2007, they recommended further ELBW infant studies needed to be done. Why? Unless I am missing something important, there is no possible justifiable reason to continue NICU ELBW experiments. What about that 2007 study?

In 2007 a Tennessee study's objective was to determine the incidence of cardio-respiratory events and abnormal c-reactive protein (CRP) levels associated with administration of single or multiple vaccines. This NICU based 239 pre-term baby study was prompted by one previously done in 1996 that showed a high incidence of apnea, bradycardia and low oxygen levels following a primary DT and whole cell pertussis (DPT) vaccine. This had already prompted a change in whole cell pertussis component to an acellular version known as TDaP in order to reduce cardio-respiratory adverse events.

After the new TDaP vaccine was introduced NICU incidences of adverse cardio-respiratory events had remained high. Authors involved in this premature baby study hypothesized there would be no similar cardio-respiratory adverse events after the TDaP. In other words their IRB was informed the proposed study would show no serious adverse events associated with TDaP. Interestingly, they also chose to determine and compare CRP levels following single TDaP injections and multiple vaccines. Contrary to their hypothesis and IRB approval elevated CRP levels were found in 70% of babies given a single vaccine and 85% of those given multiple vaccines. There were also thirty nine cardio-respiratory events. The TDaP alone accounted for 22% while 32% were attributed to multiple vaccines. A post single vaccination CRP was higher for HiB (70%), pneumococcal conjugate 54% (PCV7) than TDaP (24%) recipients, but not as high as the 80% in their multiple vaccines group. The authors concluded CRP levels can be expected to remain elevated for forty eight hours following vaccinations.

In study authors' words a minority of infants suffered a cardio-respiratory event with a presumed need for intervention. A need for intervention was identified more often in their multi-vaccinated group. A take away for parents, caregivers and doctors should be the risk for a cardio-respiratory event following a single vaccine is significant. Significance increased when multi-vaccines were given. In fact 16 % of 239 ELBW infants had a cardio-respiratory event in need of intervention. Rather than conclude this was significant they chose to use the word minority. How strange. Additionally, although gastro-esophageal reflux (GER) occurred in 17% of infants given multiple vaccines and only 7% in their single vaccine group, there was no apparent need for further comment.

As I attempted to digest this study, I was stunned by the authors reporting intraventricular brain hemorrhage (IVH) grades 3 or 4 occurred in 46 infants. The incidence in their single vaccine group was 29 out of a total of 168 (17%). In their multi-vaccine group 17 out of a total of 71 (24%) had a significant brain hemorrhage. An apparent correlation between multi-vaccine administration, abnormally high CRP levels, brain hemorrhage and reflux were not addressed in their conclusions that raises profound ethical and moral considerations and questions. Were parents of these 46 infants advised their child suffered a coincidental stroke while in the NICU, or were they advised otherwise? Is it possible authors were able to somehow statistically bury high CRP levels and a likely association with infant intraventricular hemorrhages or encephalitis?

What was the ultimate outcome for each of these 239 experimental infants, or those 13,926 in our previous study? A take away here is already unmistakable. Some significant unexpected abnormalities following vaccine administration need to be ignored or categorized as coincidental in order to continue repeating our daily increasingly dangerous vaccination program for no rational greater good. Greater good mantras can no longer be justified when researchers are able under NICU monitoring to see life threatening events with their own eyes that are as likely to occur at home in the hours or days following vaccinations. Calls to 911 are already too late and invariably futile.

Although correlation does not equate with causation, based on these studies there is no justification for continued attempts to bring premature babies up to date. Common sense should also dictate more IRB approved NICU ELBW vaccine studies are inexcusable. Apparently in this study a possible IRB shutdown was not a consideration. These studies verifying vaccine maker warnings justify withholding trust in anyone proclaiming vaccines are safe.

It is doubtful Pediatrix, Duke or Tennessee Researchers have done follow-up on their infants, who are now six to eleven years of age, in order to determine whether they remain alive and healthy. I fear some have gone on to succumb with, perhaps, one hundred deaths and thirteen hundred regressions into autism. I pray this is not the case. Not knowing eventual outcomes for these babies is an example of unjustifiable medical science. If outcomes for these NICU babies are known they should be reported, especially if they have remained healthy. Finally, I can't help wondering if there were any VAERS submissions made for any of these babies or their parents.

# 4

---

# Where To From Here?

These studies epitomize a new found way for doctors looking at their data to rationalize, exclude and then conclude things with our vaccine program are fine. There is no need to stop doing what is being done. Vaccine combinations, regardless of infant age, ethnicity and weight that have never previously been tested are safe. With this kind of medical logic coming from academic centers parents cannot trust in the veracity of doctors, especially those directly or indirectly managed by our vaccine industry. NICU's have saved countless ELBW babies. I find it shameful success in saving lives is being squandered in the name of vaccine compliance.

Not surprisingly, NICU nurse whistleblowers are slowly coming forward with information about other infant vaccine atrocity cover-ups. Before giving a vaccine every parent and healthcare worker should know something about these scientific studies, as well as, the immune and detoxification status of vaccine intended recipients. A relatively common MTHFR gene mutation may block an infant's methylation cycle making detoxification impossible. More informed healthcare workers in increasing numbers might begin to question and defy their orders. Guessing we are not doing harm going forward should become unacceptable. Guessing coincidence, rather than acknowledging consequence, is the reason we are where we are today.

When studies emerge verifying vaccines and vaccine combinations can be harmful, they cannot be ignored, in spite of abstracts and authors' conclusions. To make matters more frightening, pneumococcal conjugate (PCV7), TDaP. hemophilus influenza (HiB) and hep B vaccines given at age two months contain aluminum. Aluminum is a vaccine adjuvant used to stimulate our immune system in some unknown nonspecific fashion. Unfortunately, it just happens to be a well known nerve poison. Research authors found no need to mention aluminum. Is any amount of injected aluminum safe? Based upon a FDA researcher who studied effects of orally ingested aluminum on animals the answer according to his FDA employer, it is safe. In other words this FDA doctor is asking us to believe there is no difference between giving aluminum to rabbits by mouth or by injection. How absurd is his conclusion? Any other conclusion might lead to the removal of all aluminum from vaccines. Removal followed by a decline in SIDS and autism would be too risky to chance. A more simplified reason for doctors and nurses not doing what the CDC, ACIP, and AAP are ordering be done is to consider they are giving babies, infants, and children more than vaccines, they are injecting high doses of aluminum. Perhaps everyone should forget about names on vaccines, but remember aluminum is a known nervous system poison. Infant's innate immune systems will trap and carry aluminum directly into their brains without opposition.

No one should forget thimerosal, a combination or mercury and aluminum, was used in multi-doses vaccine vials. It had been added as a preservative, for more than 50 years and is still currently found in some multi-dose influenza and several other vaccines including TDaP. Somehow the 2001 consensus mercury could no longer be considered safe had no effect on continued use of vaccines containing aluminum. Medical experts were quick to point out thimerosal could not have been responsible for infant deaths or autism, because infants were receiving much less mercury by 2005 without a decline in SIDS or autism. This may be true, however, amounts of aluminum being given increased during this same period.

Aluminum has already been implicated in breast cancer and Alzheimer's disease. High concentrations of aluminum are being found in brains of autism victims who have died for other reasons. No one should be able to conclude aluminum is safe. No one should ever think injected aluminum is not potentially deadly. Soon readers will hear more about one injection I consider the mother of all vaccines (MOAV); namely, aluminum containing HPV vaccines named Gardasil and Cervarix. These vaccines contain more aluminum than their five nearest competitors.

It is important to keep in mind, if there is an abnormal genetic sequence, such as, the MTMFR, there is a significantly intensified potential risk for harm. In the interest of individual safety this possibility should be known well in advance of vaccination. There is also no reason to give an Afro-American child the MMR at age one when age two or three may be safer. Unsafe MMR evidence is being suppressed, but is available. If healthcare workers continue to be encouraged or possibly mandated to carry out our current practices, they should always think about injections they give may result in adverse consequences. And, at the very least, we should be prepared and willing to help a patient or parent establish a time line, if something goes wrong.

Continued healthcare worker denial there is a serious problem can no longer be tolerated. We are where we are today as a direct consequence of not thinking. Coincidence does not proceed from a known unavoidably unsafe event. Since 1986 unavoidably unsafe are words used to define vaccines. Vaccines need to be redefined by recipient beliefs as necessarily avoidable and unsafe until proven otherwise. Unbiased clear thinking medical professionals should honestly consider the possibility we have willingly participated in the creation of our growing horrific epidemics by listening to lies. Where we go from here will be determined when a critical number of doctors begin thinking and looking at their own practices. I believe they will finally see why and where we are today.

Common sense should dictate whenever there is an unexpected death or a decline in function in the hours or days following an exposure or injection, consequence rather than coincidence must become a realistic and acceptable medical explanation. Reading these NICU studies should make it impossible for doctors to continue business as usual. Many are already voicing their concerns after looking closely at correlations within their practices. Fortunately, for everyone the pendulum may be shifting with consequence replacing coincidence. When asked in the case of Nicholas' unexplained death an emergency physician proclaimed that it was not vaccine related. If he had knowledge available in TDaP's package insert his answer would have been the opposite. If this particular physician had received VAERS education he would have been more compassionate, concerned and conscientious.

European and American vaccine injury courts have acknowledged and upheld in several recent cases vaccine consequence is more likely than coincidence. In France, a man developed multiple sclerosis (MS) and in another case an infant in the United States died within hours of five vaccines. Both were ruled consequential resulting in financial compensation. Accordingly a significant paradigm shift is occurring. This swing favors the acceptance of a new belief that there is a likely cause effect relationship when a death or disability follows an event. Vaccine injections are slowly becoming acceptable explanations for serious adverse events. A cause effect truth is emerging from a myriad of adverse consequences that can no longer be contained in coincidental. Once again parents rather than medical professionals are leading the way.

There is little doubt our world belief in vaccines is crumbling. Illnesses once believed contained are re-emerging among those who have been vaccinated. This means associated viruses are mutating and are no longer recognizable by a previous artificially vaccine stimulated immune system. Recommending and giving similar vaccines becomes an exercise in futility. All Harvard and Princeton students surviving an outbreak of mumps at twenty years of age may already have a new memory with a natural ability to ward off future strains. Wasting money on reminding our immune system of old invaders serves no useful medial purpose. The good news is new invaders come in without aluminum, mercury, formaldehyde, MSG, neomycin, polysorbitol, yeast or sequences of foreign human embryo, monkey or bovine, potentially carcinogenic, DNA. The bad news is vaccine makers are facing a problem their old products are becoming obsolete. How many times can you sell an ineffective product to the same recipient?

Perhaps it is time for wise people to stop, look and listen. Parents, caregiver and healthcare workers can no longer ignore the flashing warning lights. A runaway vaccine train has already plowed through other poorly protected crossings. A growing list of honest scientific studies and whistleblowers internal to our CDC and vaccine manufacturers is emerging.

In the interim it is time for the American College of Emergency Physicians to step up and become involved by reporting every infant and child coming into an emergency department who has died without reason or become ill within four weeks of receiving a vaccine. There is no time for making further excuses for not doing so. Informed ACEP leadership cannot shrink from this simple task. Reporting vaccine suspicions is a mandatory law. Ignoring clinical impressions is the hallmark feature of a bad physician. When good emergency physicians hear hoof beats, they think about zebras rather than horses. Vaccine adverse events are emergency room zebras.

Manufacturers and NICU researchers have provided enough evidence for most to conclude there is something inherently wrong with our current approach to preventing childhood illnesses. It is now apparent attempting prevention is far worse than most illnesses we are trying to preclude. It is already evident vaccines are responsible for emerging more serious illnesses. A simple example might be Guillain-Barré Syndrome (GBS). GBS has been known to follow vaccinations for forty years, but only in the past several years have GBS influenza vaccine victims received compensation awards. Vaccine inserts have listed GBS warnings since 1976. GBS vaccine victim compensation has dramatically risen annually since inclusion reaching more than fifty million dollars this past year.

# 5

---

# What about the Precautionary Principle?

In 1998 scientists, ethicists, lawyers and activists convened at the Wingspread Conference in Madison, Wisconsin. Attendees rallied behind a proactive position called the Precautionary Principle. This coming together was a reaction against growing scandals associated with injuries from synthetic chemicals, pesticides, insecticides, tobacco, asbestos and vaccines. This principle represented a dramatic departure from traditional thinking by reducing requirements necessary for proving cause and effect relationships.

Under the Precautionary Principle suspicion of a danger without absolute proof becomes the new premise for taking some form of action. More specifically it means a shift in the burden of proof. When an activity raises threats of harm to human health or the environment, precautionary measures should be taken even if some cause effect relationships are not fully established scientifically. In this context the proponent of an activity, other than the public, should bear the full burden of proof. The process of applying the Precautionary Principle must be open, informed and democratic and must include potentially affected parties. It must also involve an examination of the full range of alternatives including no action.

Manufacturers and researchers recognizing threats of vaccine harm to human health can no longer be held harmless. They both must bear a full burden of proof for justifying their own continued activities when issues of cause and effect are becoming more obvious than ever. Continuing to do nothing when the public good is at stake is unacceptable.

I am convinced our IOM in 2003 had enough information to justify issuance of a vaccine warning in the name of The Precautionary Principle that certain vaccines, combinations and their ingredients are dangerous. When a reasonable suspicion exists concerning a product's safety continued use of that product cannot be condoned. The onus for safety must be shifted to makers rather than require a victim to prove injury was caused by that product. There was no reason our IOM failed to take action other than perpetuating indemnification and continuing a cover-up. For our IOM to go on to recommend there was no need for further vaccine safety studies was preposterous.

There should also be a suspicion the original details of our CDC's Georgia MMR vaccine Afro-American study were disclosed to members. Although this is at best speculation, in light of a CDC whistleblower's revelations about a sudden internal urgency for cleansing the original study findings that showed an increased MMR autism risk for one year old Afro-American children, it may not be an unreasonable proposition. Imagine IOM members being told the MMR vaccine given to Afro-Americans was associated with a dramatic increased risk for autism.

In the IOM aftermath something occurred that may be important. A prominent member Dr. Bernadine Healy, a highly respected cardiologist, came forward. She alluded to some internal turmoil in discussions about vaccine dangers and the public good. Rather than be truthful and possibly undermine existing vaccine science, there was an apparent agreed upon code of silence? Dr. Healy, among others, could not have been happy with this outcome. By agreeing to an interview a former head of our NIH was acknowledging overall emphasis had been on protecting vaccine policy. IOM had likely become even more tainted by failing to recommend additional vaccine safety testing.

It would be fair to say, neither Dr. Healy nor Sharyl Attkisson, a journalist, who conducted her interview, received any praise for their respective candor. No attempt has been made to do either a study to compare the health of unvaccinated and vaccinated children, or to identify a susceptible infant population. As a result, a one size fits all vaccine policy has seemingly remained untouched, in spite of mounting contrary evidence. IOM members chose to do nothing, but vaccine makers may have felt their protective bubble was at risk.

Perhaps, knowing there may have been genuine IOM concern and flaws within the law protecting them, vaccine makers sought added legal protection. Their path would lead to our Supreme Court where a favorable majority vote added further protection from vaccine injury liability claims. Safety evidence presented to Supreme Court Justices must have been impressive, although a favorable outcome with support coming from President Obama was no surprise. Vaccine makers got everything they wanted. A minority Justice made it clear she had heard vaccine safety evidence and in her opinion she stated vaccines have been and continue to be unavoidably unsafe.

Many physicians, researchers, lawyers, academic scientists and whistle blowers have come forward to expose reasons why an unavoidably unsafe moniker was attached to vaccines without reference to growing numbers and an increasingly congested vaccine timetable. At a time when our Supreme Court majority voted in favor of no manufacturer liability for damages inflicted by vaccines, including their toxic adjuvant ingredients, our vaccine makers must have experienced a sigh of relief. Imagine how powerful this industry has become, when on one hand it admits to the possibility of vaccine damage and death, and on the other hand, requests and is granted unlimited product liability protection. With current outbreaks of mumps, pertussis and measles almost exclusively among individuals fully vaccinated, our Supreme Court apparently agreed vaccines do not need to be either safe or effective.

An answer to this question may be found in 2002. Vaccine makers and our CDC needed a scientific study to prove there was no possible link between vaccines and autism. A paper had previously appeared in the literature in 1999 which suggested there was a possible correlation between MMR vaccinations and autism. This CDC sponsored study conducted in Denmark and published in 2002 that allegedly disproved any possible link became their overdue proof. Quickly this study's fraudulent process and conclusions began to unravel forcing vaccine makers to deal with the inevitable fallout. A CDC funded study published in a scientific journal and our New York Times was a fake.

Our mainstream media went silent concerning charges made against the study's author, Dr. Poul Thorsen, for fraud, embezzlement and money laundering followed by his indictment in Denmark. His Danish study authorized and paid for by our CDC to provide proof that would end a growing vaccine controversy was statistically unraveling. Key doctors with CDC ties and network affiliations forgot about trying to defend this questionable study. Rather than support their products vaccine makers chose instead to launch a counter offensive. Vaccine makers would choose to aggressively pursue and attempt to discredit vaccine dissenters, while seeking added legal protection.

Our vaccine industry saw a need to strategically fortify its position. The timing was perfect. Major media outlets had already lost major advertising sponsors, tobacco and alcohol leaving a significant income void. Pharmaceutical and chemical companies were financially able and ready to step up with their own fiscal clout. With a few disclaimers about a possibility of death or disability at the beginning of their drug advertisements directed at viewers, miracle cures were promised. All viewers would need to do would be to ask their doctors for a prescription. Celebrities and paid actors marketing their products directly to viewers was a bold step, although gaining actual control of network media would be their overall strategy. Broadcast journalists might think twice before airing carefully corroborated but potentially damaging vaccine and chemical stories. Silencing highly paid network spokespeople could be accomplished by controlling the purse strings.

Withholding potentially damaging vaccine information might be construed by station managers to be in the interest of public good, rather than their own. No one selfishly in control of our media could have foreseen there would be continued erosion. Social media impact had been immensely underestimated. Dangerous stories promulgated by rebel non-corporate journalists and lay witnesses were banding together to tell their own versions creating a growing breach that was getting out of their control.

Vaccine industry and research warnings, if not broadcast, would do no harm, especially with Presidential and Supreme Court blessings.

There is little doubt history was again repeating itself. Vaccine maker executives had another industry as an example of what should be done. Forestalling could be extraordinarily profitable, if our medical profession and media could be controlled. With no liability there would be no reason for anyone to attempt shifting a burden of vaccine safety proof to the makers.

What happened during those years between Thorsen's Danish study, a meeting of our IOM and other events, ultimately leading to our Supreme Court's ruling, is of interest, starting with Dr. Andrew Wakefield. Wakefield had published an IRB, peer reviewed 1999 study which suggested there was a MMR autism link. Attempted CDC studies disproving any link had failed, so attention needed to be directed at Wakefield, if it was going to remain vaccine business as usual. Pharmaceutical industry paid pro-vaccine bloggers aggressively went to work on quelling growing parental vaccine discontent on social media, while vaccine makers with help from traditional medicine and the media targeted Wakefield.

# 6

---

# Lessons from our Past

A famous physicist tinkering with atoms was responsible for creating our knowledge of atomic energy. The Atomic bomb some might consider was a logical consequence of his brilliance. It has been reported Einstein said, if he knew about the destruction it would cause, he might have chosen to become a shoemaker. Likewise, widespread tinkering with our human immune system has unleashed irreparable damage to humanity and our human blueprint, perhaps, precipitating far more destruction than releasing atomic energy over two cities.

Tinkering with vaccines began more than 200 years ago. Dairy workers exposed to cowpox disease did not appear to get smallpox. This led to deliberately exposing non-dairy workers to unknown cowpox ingredients with serious adverse consequences, including deaths. Further tinkering led to a more sophisticated scratch vaccination. Perhaps, if quarantine and sanitation were understood, vaccine related deaths could have been reduced, even if vaccines turned out to be useless. There was a degree of insanity contained in subsequent destructive medical and public health smallpox vaccine mandates that would have been revealed, if only someone in authority with power had intervened by reading available contrary literature.

Rather than believe those tinkering for profit actually knew what they were doing there was scientific evidence that for many people smallpox vaccines would be more deadly than the disease. Initially, a few knowledgeable individuals resisted then others totally refused to take this vaccine. Communities soon followed by an entire city refused with no reported cases of smallpox. Invoking sanitation and quarantine measures provided proof smallpox was preventable and vaccines were both unsafe and dangerous. In a 1789 publication titled *Vaccination*, released during a smallpox outbreak in England, the author singled out British military personnel offered proof vaccines were not helpful. Both soldiers and sailors had been given mandatory vaccinations. Not surprising, soldiers continued to develop disease at a rate similar to England's general population, whereas smallpox among sailors was more than double. The author concluded that an absence of reasonable shipboard sanitation was responsible. Data collected in a registry over a forty year period regarding this vaccine was contained in the author's title *Vaccinations dangerous and useless*. His data was presented to Parliament in 1789. Health Ministry members would not agree. A governmental precedent was established to ignore any future studies suggesting vaccines were both useless and dangerous.

Since the introduction of vaccines the principle of homeopathy has been a tenet. If a suspected disease cause could be diluted practically out of existence, it might be safely given to prevent a similar illness. Continued tinkering led to introduction of live, dead and attenuated viral and bacterial versions of an actual illness. By using an environment for culture containing human embryonic or animal DNA and RNA new vaccines emerged from laboratories containing antibiotics, heavy metals, formaldehyde and additional ingredients including contaminants to enhance stimulation of a human antibody immune response. Many of these foreign DNA gene sequences and toxic ingredients now known to be unsafe have remained in use for more than fifty years. Many have become part of our human blueprint not necessarily for any good. If there had been adequate testing we would have known better. Today we are witness to these vaccine consequences. Our sophisticated immune systems react to practically everything not recognized creating widespread confusion and antibodies directed against both good and bad.

In 2018 so much more is known about genomes, genetic mapping, gene editing and repair. What might have been proclaimed victories over childhood illnesses in greater good's name has instead planted seeds for current and future immune and neurological system disarray and destruction. In tinkering processes there is no doubt we have created innumerable destructive genetically controlled diseases. These epigenetic diseases will be passed on unless repair is possible. The good news is repairing genes is possible. This new multi-billion dollar industry may someday be able to undo tinkering damage for those still alive or about to be born. Creating future pure genetic vaccines without contamination or adjuvant risks may also be possible. Meanwhile, there is considerable bad news. We must bring an end to what vaccine makers have been primitively doing and have these same manufacturers participate in paying for the related damage.

Understanding who is to blame at this moment may help parents decide if anyone can be trusted. Moral and ethical principles must become weapons against destruction by forcefully making their way to the forefront. If I had known I was destined to become a vendor or provider rather than a physician, I would likely have chosen another career. Medicine today is not what it once was, in spite of contrary claims. America is spending more on healthcare per person than any country on our planet with thirty two countries remaining ahead in terms of health and longevity. Premature deaths from opioid overdoses have played a medically sanctioned role, but are not a significant factor when compared to medical and surgical induced deaths. More people die in America annually from medications and mistakes than in our last three wars combined. Doctors have become pharmaceutical rather than medical providers. Vaccines have caused far more damage than good. Recently, my thinking was refreshed when a mother visiting from Sweden, where vaccines are not mandated, brought her daughter into my clinic with a classic chickenpox rash. After confirming her suspicion was correct this child's mother was actually elated with the diagnosis and refused any pharmaceutical treatment.

It is time for me to try to help what I consider a once noble profession from being dragged down further by pharmaceutical greed and corruption. My beliefs have been defined and refined by interpreting what I have been told and what I have actually seen over fifty years. Simply put, money has become a sole governing factor in medical decision making. Iatrogenesis is playing a more prominent role in medicine than imaginable. I can't help but feel sorry for younger doctors, who only believe what they continue to be told. Our current plight is an example of leadership failure. Allowing our pharmaceutical vaccine industry to take over infant, childhood and adult medicine is disgraceful. Lessons about mistakes taken from our distant past should never be ignored otherwise they will repeat, if patterns are not recognized. Trying to eradicate by waging war against childhood illnesses with vaccines has become far more destructive to humans than those same viruses.

Dr. Ignaz Semmelweis was a physician in Vienna around 1840. He recognized a pattern surrounding deaths following labor and delivery at his maternity hospital which differed significantly from a facility run only by midwives. He realized mothers-to-be had become so frightened they would choose to have their babies on the street rather than in his maternity ward. Postpartum fevers followed by death convinced Semmelweis that his doctors were doing something different than nearby midwives. Semmelweis determined a likely cause by observations alone. He saw doctors going from the morgue to his delivery room. Deductive reasoning forced him to conclude whatever was causing deaths was coming with his doctors, because midwives did not do autopsies.

Hand washing before delivery brought about a dramatic reduction in puerperal fever deaths. Lister, Koch and Pasteur had not yet come on the scene with a germ hypothesis for disease. Semmelweis' hypothesis doctors were responsible was treated with disdain by traditional medicine. Iatrogenic deaths were not possible. Doctors were too noble to be a cause. Semmelweis was dismissed from his position. A short time later, at age forty seven he died in an asylum most likely from wound infection. His life had deteriorated following his dismissal and ongoing professional scorn. Iatrogenesis in his maternity ward came to an end because younger doctors witnessing a dramatic shift began to routinely wash their hands.

Perhaps there are good lessons from our past. Unfortunately new contrary information does not necessarily go over well. Although other traditional doctors could have recognized a pattern, they did not. The rate from child birth death was reduced from fifty per cent to one percent. Traditional medicine, not believing in the possibility doctors were carriers of disease, turned their backs. Fortunately, some did not do so and it would make all the difference. One of those who refused to turn his back more than 200 years later was Andrew Wakefield.

# 7

## The Road Not Taken

Parents, caregivers and physicians now find themselves at a critical cross road patrolled by medical experts, media spokespeople and law makers directing them not to choose a road less taken. If there is hesitancy or a decision not to follow the path of least resistance, parents will be warned of both obvious and unseen obstacles and consequences for their wrong choices. I am here to say there is no wrong choice. Freewill by definition dictates there is always a choice. Protecting freedom in the name of babies' lives must become the new mantra.

At this juncture evidence for the true safety of our most traveled vaccine road does not exist. In fact, evidence is mounting vaccine combinations and their ingredients are not safe and less importantly they are ineffective. Vaccines are in many cases similar to improvised road side devices. Victims may receive devastating injuries and live, while others die without evidence of injury. Without causal evidence growing epidemics afflicting all ages paralleling vaccine use and our vaccine schedule must be attributed to what we continue to do wrong, or not do at all. Statistical support for this statement is known. Members of our medical profession, rather than stand in unison singing a vaccination anthem, should separate and silently begin protesting. Physicians saying no to unsafe vaccines and adjuvants in the name of babies' lives are a far more intelligent next step.

Those of us in defiance will begin sending a single clear message that babies' lives matter more than those of our vaccine makers. Until there is a controlled study providing incontrovertible evidence today's vaccine industry is not responsible for infant and childhood sudden deaths and grave neurological injuries and deterioration in all ages, we cannot be mandated to blindly continue to obey. Without an honest safety study, there will be a rapidly growing number of doctors rightfully willing to provide vaccine medical exemptions for children of parents and caregivers not choosing to be ordered to take a road most traveled or to ignore flashing light warnings. This free choice path based on informed consent will not be easy. I am prepared to take the risk to defend this right as a doctor, father, grandfather and great grandfather. I firmly believe we would never have gotten into our current toxic epidemic dilemma, if our health profession had been more vigilant and less compliant. If doctors had insisted on knowing real dangers associated with procedures, drugs, vaccines and their complicated ingredients and had obtained informed consent before prescribing or injecting and had agreed to report adverse events, we would not find ourselves at our current point of no return.

The vaccine pro-choice movement will be met with deep-pocket resistance some may consider too dangerous to oppose. Already pro-choice movement members have sustained unexplained, but not coincidental deaths. Doctors and journalists in the ranks of this movement are being singled out for elimination. Casualty lists will continue to grow, but there will be new resistors swelling our ranks. Talk rather than walk from legislators will cost them their jobs. Those resorting to promoting statewide mandates may suffer more severe fates due to their acceptance of what some may construe as bad science and blood money.

Vaccine benefit has been transformed into a healthcare disciple run religion and business making finding a flaw in either an unacceptable outcome. As a result, layer upon layer of medical, industrial and legal half truths have been used to justify an unsafe continuation and escalation. Consider for a moment the sheer stupidity of doctors telling mothers-to-be to get mercury containing flu shots, but not eat mercury carrying fish. It's even harder to understand how a doctor considered an expert can say ingested methyl mercury in fish is more dangerous than injected ethyl mercury in vaccines. Each should know better. At least when mercury is orally consumed it can either be excreted or if it enters the blood stream, depending on amount, it can be eliminated by healthy detoxification pathways. This is not the case when mercury and aluminum are injected. Should anyone be surprised mothers with mercury containing dental fillings are at nine-fold greater risk of bearing an infant destined for autism.

At a time when pregnant mothers-to-be are being advised to get flu shots and TDaP boosters they are actually being told by doctors with each pregnancy they need mercury and aluminum contained in each of these vaccines. Infant grandparents are being told a similar story, if they wish to visit. Should it not be surprising our fetal death rate in America is so high? There has also been an alarming increase in maternal deaths. Perhaps those investigators at Duke University are on to something much bigger, but cannot visualize or even imagine the magnitude of the problem created by condoning wholesale multi-vaccines. Semmelweis without vaccine maker support may have drawn another conclusion; namely, iatrogenesis.

At a time when brains of young autism spectrum disorder (ASD) victims are being found to contain larger than could have ever been expected deposits of aluminum, especially, among boys, should we act surprised? When a vaccine expert tells us ethyl mercury is safe should we not be dumbfounded? If this same individual tells us aluminum is safe for ELBW babies should we be astonished? If he chooses to say otherwise he might have to conclude he is in some way responsible for what is happening. Experts professing vaccines are safe for every infant cannot rationally be prepared to defend the adjuvants, ingredients and contaminants without pointing a finger to some other factor. No wise person needs to invoke unknown factors when known poisons are routinely being administered to our children. Researchers may come up with increasing use of hormones in fertility drugs as brain damaging, but a look at Mississippi data may harbor evidence changing that hypothesis.

I do not mean to single out any particular doctors who are willing to be continued apologists for our vaccine industry. Contrary evidence suggests they have chosen to single themselves out by making safety and effectiveness proclamations. If these same individuals were not featured media spokespeople walking a tightrope between medicine and vaccine makers, they probably would not even stand out. When they reap enormous financial benefit from creating their own vaccine, at best, they are no better than Wakefield, perhaps much worse.

Vaccine adjuvants have acted as neurological poisons. Both mercury and aluminum get into infant brains adversely affecting the ability of non-neuron microglia to do their jobs. Microglia carrying aluminum can slip directly into an infant's central nervous system. Microglia containing aluminum is also being found in the brains of younger and younger victims of Alzheimer's disease (AD). Is it possible AD is actually being caused by vaccine practices over the past thirty to forty years? The answer should be a resounding yes! Tinkering and tampering with our human immune system has wrought unaccounted for damages now appearing in all ages. Vaccine inventors and makers may ultimately be held accountable by mothers of babies whose lives' matter.

After extensive research one of those mothers exposed mercury's neurotoxicity resulting in a decision favoring its removal from vaccines by writing a book revealing similarities between mercury damaged children and those with autistic behaviors. Mercury would be removed with the stipulation that mercury containing vaccines could still be given to newborns, infants and children until existing three to four year supplies were depleted or expired. In other words no recall would be necessary. Meanwhile vaccine manufacturers continued to use aluminum and ship their thimerosal products to developing countries. As seemingly ridiculous as this scenario may seem, not surprisingly manufacturers continued to proclaim mercury is safe at a time when those vaccinated in these same developing nations are experiencing a five-fold increase in pervasive developmental disorders (PDD) when compared with unvaccinated children.

Years earlier a manufacturer of DDT, reeling in defeat after another woman exposed its danger in a book titled *The Silent Spring* continued to proclaim their product was safe. Shipments outside the United States were not interrupted. Perhaps, this was a marketing ploy, because they were already in possession of a successor product known as Glyphosate (Round-Up). Similarly vaccine manufacturers were somehow equally successful by managing to resume marketing mercury containing influenza vaccines. Pro-mercury medical experts trying to prove its safety pointed to a peer reviewed study which showed infant's injected with ethyl mercury had no mercury in blood samples a month later.

Once again, a well known expert, offered his opinion this study was proof infants could readily detoxify ethyl mercury. Where did it go? No mercury was found in infant urine or stool. Mercury had apparently by-passed possible detoxification pathways by going directly into infant brains. With the blessings of Dr. Paul Offit, a known nerve toxic agent was being deliberately injected into infants destined to be deposited in their nervous tissues where maximum harm would be possible. Is it possible this expert really didn't know the ultimate destination of the missing mercury? Is it possible this study had been approved in advance by an IRB? If true, were parents advised of the potential risks associated with this infant mercury injection experiment? Were mercury injected babies given a lifelong guarantee there would be no neurological damage? This study reinforces actual harm being done by doctors choosing parental coercion without any guarantees of short or long term infant safety or long term follow up. This continued practice is illegal. Unethical and immoral implications have already been well established.

During 2016, when supplies of mercury free influenza vaccines were depleted, California's health commissioner gave her approval for doctors to use mercury containing shots for pregnant women. One day, while covering a family physician's practice, a pregnant woman came with a prescription from her obstetrician for a flu shot. Before ordering, I asked her to read the package insert's section on possible adverse events. Although a heightened risk of miscarriage was not listed, based upon the amount of mercury alone, she chose to pass. As a result, I have never been invited back to this office. I had done something unthinkable by exposing this young mother and her baby to the manufacturer's warnings, rather than mercury. The price I paid was small. It became another important lesson. It was pale in comparison to what happened to Semmelweis and Wakefield.

When there is mounting evidence vaccines given during pregnancy have been associated with increased spontaneous abortions, does any of this continue to make sense? There is no reason to give a fetus a chick embryo cultured flu vaccine, possibly containing mercury, when vaccine manufacturers do not recommend their product for infants less than six months. What are vaccine manufacturers hiding? What are doctors thinking? Regardless, with new information this vaccine is also ineffective due to a processing mutation the very act of giving it becomes unethical and immoral. Doesn't it?

If scientists and state health commissioners are allowed to tell physicians what to do, we may have reached a last straw doctor scenario. When health professionals are being herded into ignoring vaccine dangers and submitting to the will of our CDC, ACIP, AAP and vaccine makers there is a monumental problem. Doctors are becoming pharmaceutical providers easily replaceable by far less trained mid-level providers with prescription writing licenses. Physicians' moral and ethical obligations not to do possible harm or impose personal, religious or vaccine beliefs on patients are being overridden and are now becoming the new norm. Can continued physician coercion and parental vaccine compliance demands become the acceptable standard? I say doctors must retake control.

Accepting healthcare workers beliefs that override contrary information presently available in vaccine inserts, in scientific articles and on social media has now become an either or issue. Can any doctor receiving financial gain from vaccinating a majority of their infant population be trusted? Can any healthcare corporation or organization receiving money directly or indirectly from our vaccine industry act in the best interests of their patients, or employees? Can any vaccine inventor who brags about vaccinating his own children as a proof for safety be trusted? Can I as a physician who had my own five children vaccinated be trusted?

Not long ago a Minnesota based healthcare organization fired fifty nurses for refusing our most recent ineffective and possibly dangerous influenza vaccine. With a strong likelihood vaccinated people are still getting influenza illnesses, this termination policy makes absolutely no sense. I am hopeful these nurses will get their jobs back including any accruing financial damages. If any nurses agreeing to a flu shot, as a condition for employment, develop Guillain-Barré Syndrome or multiple sclerosis, is it likely their healthcare corporation employer will share in payments for damages? If I were an attorney, I would probably choose to defend those who refuse, rather than the vaccine bullies.

With a recent yet unconfirmed report from Santa Barbara, California of nine deaths from our most recent flu outbreak, should it be any surprise eight are reported to have received the flu vaccine? Would they be alive today, if they refused? Far more deadly hospital acquired infections should be of greatest concern. A published article from Boston confirmed during the last Swine flu outbreak hospitalized children, who died ostensibly from flu virus, actually died from hospital acquired Methicillin resistant staphylococcal (MRSA) pneumonia. Hospitalization may be far more dangerous than influenza.

Robert Frost's poem *The Road Less Taken* is poignant. He points out in this and other works his horse, a creature of habit, is of the programmed opinion, there is only one way to go. The one holding his reins concludes, after taking an alternative road less traveled, it has made all the difference. Semmelweis took a road less traveled. Dr. Andrew Wakefield chose a road less traveled. Parents exercising informed consent are holding the reins with a right to take a road less traveled. Doctors cannot be allowed to remain in control especially when there is vaccination money at stake. A pediatrician in Minnesota recently took a less traveled road by revealing giving parents a right to say no has cost his practice more than $1,000,000 a year. He is also on record stating his unvaccinated patients are his healthiest. Saying no to either a doctor or horse is not easy. Parents must take those reins by withholding informed consent based upon what manufacturers' state in their vaccine inserts. Pediatricians in Oregon and Minnesota have seen a forest once blocked by a tree. More saying no to vaccines combined with more medical exemptions will result in more good than harm.

# 8

---

# Getting Things into Better Perspective

As a physician approaching his 50th year in medical practice, I have been witness to ongoing compromises and excuses likely contributing to our current epidemics of death and disability. In the process I have become ashamed of failing to act sooner. If doctors practicing emergency medicine had dutifully reported every serious event suspected to be temporally related to a vaccine or listened to parental concern and suspicion, we would have reached this critical point in time twenty five years ago. The sheer volume of ignored adverse events would have forced an honest and transparent re-evaluation of safety issues surrounding what is being injected into our newborns, infants, children, teenagers and adults long before our country's millennium. If every emergency, urgent care, family and pediatric physician had been informed there was a possible inherent danger in proliferating vaccine numbers and combinations, I believe we all would have agreed to work in concert by participating in our VAERS process. We were never told. If our FDA concern at that time was an absence of documented safety, reporting suspected adverse events would have led to new safety measures, rather than allow what has been continuing to unfold.

As a once full-time emergency physician, neither I nor my colleagues, were ever told our role in a passive vaccine surveillance system, much less its importance. Infant deaths and illnesses in the hours and days following a vaccine or vaccine cocktail were all considered coincidental. None of us had been given reason to believe otherwise. Instead something terribly wrong has been allowed to unfold, supposedly in the name of achievable childhood illness prevention, rather than safety. Manufacturers have provided us with warnings, however, more often than not they have gone unnoticed for a number of reasons. Foremost is a fear of increased parental hesitancy or refusal with full risk disclosure. Next, our adverse event reporting process was relatively unknown among physicians, or if known, was too cumbersome and time consuming. Recent attempts to bring our reporting process into an electronic age have been abandoned due to a larger than anticipated and unacceptable increase in adverse event reports. A third, and in my opinion, most troubling reason, is the entire vaccine issue has been taken out of any physician decision-making process by heavily backed pharmaceutical financially inspired medical experts, insurance companies, media personalities and legislative mandates.

Physicians and other health care providers have become recipients of financial rewards for vaccine promotion and compliance. Physicians are now being told to ignore what is becoming more obvious or risk the potential consequences. Monetary and legal implications of even a slight admission vaccines may be dangerous, in spite of their immunity, terrify both manufacturers and my own profession. Mothers accustomed to trusting their children to pediatricians are also frightened at any thought they are being mislead into believing no harm can come from five simultaneously given vaccines. If something happens in the aftermath, denial will follow as night follows day. Nevertheless, concerned parents and nurses and some doctors are resisting vaccine mandates by their growing knowledge and open defiance.

These pro-choice doctors will likely receive investigation warning threats from medical licensing boards, if they choose to speak out or provide vaccine exemptions for any reason. At the same time manufacturers have openly admitted to ineffectiveness and risks associated with their products our health profession is receiving financial rewards for obedience by not breaking ACIP and AAP imposed rules. They are also being warned of possible loss of license for actions considered contrary to the public good.

Several years ago California state legislators passed SB 277 mandating vaccine compliance for public school attendance. In order to assure passage doctors were allowed to provide necessary medical exemptions. Due to a reported increase in children receiving physician exemptions new pharmaceutical inspired legislation will attempt to further restrict or abolish this provision. Media personnel have described doctor medical exemptions as nothing more than a vaccine mandate loophole in need of closure. If a physician makes an informed decision to complete an exemption form or write a letter, it could be asking for trouble. A Los Angeles Times reporter characterized doctors offering medical exemptions as mercenary. In other words, unless there is no charge for an office visit a doctor is selling medical exemptions. Perhaps, some ethicists and moralists would consider this healthier, do no harm medicine, than doctors selling vaccines. Maybe this same journalist is unaware selling vaccines has become a standard of care and is far more lucrative than providing a much needed medical exemption.

Before its too late for doctors to practice do no vaccine harm medicine every physician should consider providing a reasonable number of pro bono medical exemptions. Our job is to respect and protect our patients from harm regardless of what we are being told by an industry that is out of control, a CDC that sells $4 billion worth of vaccines each year and journalists being told what to say in order to keep their jobs. Reporting every possible adverse vaccine event and offering medical exemptions may be our only way to bring things back into perspective. Exemptions for a growing list of medically indicated reasons may represent a way for physicians to regain respect and control of their own practices.

More specifically, due to harm this vaccine is causing worldwide every child approaching their teenage years should be offered a complimentary Gardasil or Cervarix medical exemption upon request. Or better yet, doctors concerned after reading or hearing about Gardasil harm being reported in Denmark, France, Columbia and Japan should begin to warn families. Proactively attempting to protect teenage girls and boys is really a precept of physician privilege. Before doing so physicians, who are also parents, should first consult with their spouses or partners to discuss and decide what they should do for their own teenagers. Informed doctors signing informed consents for their daughters and sons must be prepared to take full responsibility for the consequences of any decisions made.

It is doubtful more than half of California physicians understand SB277. Children, including those of doctors, can be given Gardasil or Cervarix without parental consent. In my opinion injection without signed consent should be considered assault and battery. Gardasil with aluminum cannot be considered safe. Also, due to evidence Afro-American children may represent a vulnerable subset they should all be given first year MMR vaccine exemptions. No infants, especially those characterized as ELBW, should ever be given multi-vaccines. Supported by published peer reviewed NICU studies, CDC whistleblower reports and manufacturer warnings automatic medical exemptions must be used to stop continued wholesale administration of NICU vaccine cocktails until further animal safety studies, other than by Wakefield, are completed. Justifiable reasons for many medical exemptions will become evident, if an adequate history containing allergic symptoms or minimal adverse event signs appeared following any round of previous vaccinations.

Based upon NICU studies no parent of an ELBW infant should allow their baby to be experimented upon by vaccine researchers. In fact, NICU pediatricians should provide medical exemptions for all ELBW infants in their care, or be prepared to pay for the possible consequences, if anything goes wrong in attempting to bring these fragile human beings up to date. Lastly, our entire vaccine schedule boils down to a violation of human rights. Every child who has had any unusual post-vaccination adverse event deserves a medical exemption preventing use of any previously given injections.

Rather than provide risk education for physicians back in the 1980's or even attempt to do so now, total emphasis has instead been placed on vague health and practice benefits, rather than proven patient safety. My own physician surveys have revealed most doctors and nurses today do not understand either vaccine related illnesses or possible consequences of a failure to recognize one. In fact an emergency medicine article on causes for childhood seizures made no reference to vaccines. At that same time I received an FDA email warning stating seizures were twice as likely when measles, mumps, rubella vaccines included a chickenpox component (MMRV). To me this was an outright admission MMR's were causing seizures.

The total number of post MMR and MMRV seizures five years ago was unknown. If no nurse or physician suspected a vaccine given several days or weeks earlier was responsible, it would go unreported even if a parent insisted a vaccine had caused the seizure. When I questioned those study authors, I received no response. When I offered to write an article on serious vaccine adverse events, I was advised not to bother. I was told it would not be a good fit. I have since been told our AMA leaders are saying, as far as vaccines are concerned, not to even bother going there. Medical journals and our AMA depend on pharmaceutical money. Nothing considered offensive should disturb the flow of dollars.

The much heralded elimination of chickenpox has now been a consequential cause of our rapidly growing epidemic of shingles. Naturally acquired immunity from having had chickenpox as a child is no longer being reinforced by exposures to actual cases of illness. As a result, even those with tinker free immune systems are confronting a far more dangerous disease. In spite of a shingles vaccine designed to fill a created void, results have been quite opposite with far greater suffering and death. I question how this has been for the greater good. Perhaps we should be asking whose? In order to get things back into perspective we need to allow for a return of natural chickenpox outbreaks before shingles begins striking the brains and eyes of younger and younger age groups.

Five or so years ago sudden infant death and autism warnings appeared on diphtheria, tetanus and pertussis package inserts. This should have been sufficient to scare doctors and parents vaccine suit-proof manufacturers are admitting these events are factual possibilities. At the same time almost everyone else in authority was saying there is no link between these diseases and vaccines. It seems preposterous to say DPT can, but doesn't have any adverse consequences. This conclusion is simply not believable. Nicholas' mother now knows brief illnesses suffered following prior vaccinations were harbingers of things to come. An exemption for Nicholas would now seem to have been rational and, in retrospect, absolutely essential and acceptable. With mounting evidence of dreadful events coming from NICU experiments, a time to say an informed consent "no thank you" is at hand. It is already too late for many.

More than twenty years ago a young pediatric investigator pointed to a significant number of possible DPT related infant deaths and injuries only to be booed and ridiculed by his physician audience. Likely shattered and subsequently shackled, he went silent. If his knowledge and evidence had been accepted as a *precautionary principle* warning, things might have been allowed to change. Instead he was categorized as a scaremonger. This grave newly associated consequential adverse event, if published, might have been another turning point. Many mothers, who suspected DPT was the cause of their normally developing child's regression, like those of Chris and Philip, would have come forward with a chance to force manufacturers to prove their DPT was not the cause.

Possibly intellectually honest physicians might have been forced to pay closer attention. It did not happen. Instead, immediately ensuing fevers and prolonged sleeping illnesses experienced by Chris and Philip were considered normal by their pediatricians. A reasonably intelligent doctor should have recognized encephalitis, an inflammatory brain illness, could be a fatal or debilitating illness. Package inserts already listed encephalitis as a serious adverse event. Quietly manufacturers replaced their suspected encephalitis cause, the cellular pertussis component, with a new acellular variation. Rather than admit and then confront parents of unknown numbers of DPT vaccine damaged children our liability free industry deliberately chose to go in the opposite direction. Replacing DPT with TDaP did not result in an improvement as previously shown by NICU researchers. Adverse events had long been a concern for vaccine makers.

Manufacturers had already decided actuarial liability associated with their vaccine products was simply too great to remain profitable. During the 1976 Swine flu scare our vaccine industry had been asked to create a vaccine combining a swine component with their current seasonal flu product. In exchange manufacturers asked for and were granted indemnification for any harm their combined product might cause. The National Influenza Immunization Program (NIIP) spearheaded a drive to vaccinate as many individuals of all ages as possible, in spite the fact, Swine flu was not being found outside of Fort Dix, New Jersey.

A politically inspired campaign ended six months later. Evidence suggested more harm than good was occurring. Bad outcomes were initially attributed to coincidence by network media. It was reported after vaccination three older men died in the same office on the same day. Vaccine makers without liability for their hastily created product had done their job. Deaths, autoimmune disease and neurological injuries, such as Guillain-Barré Syndrome, were a small price to pay for a potential, but never realized politically inspired pandemic.

It might be fair to say, vaccine makers learned an important lesson in scrambling to create what the government wanted. Stopping further vaccine production might work better than trying to prove their products were safe became a central theme for a new corporate strategy. Perhaps, not knowing continued production carried more adverse risks for babies and infants than benefits, our governmental response was, "Please don't stop production, you can have whatever you want." A well prepared vaccine industry knew fears of a widespread epidemic of lock jaw, if the tetanus vaccine was discontinued, would trump any inherent danger. Our vaccine industry threat was taken seriously so something had to be done to avoid a recurrence of plagues.

Vaccine manufacturers had found a way to mitigate their immediate and future risks. In order to continue business as usual in 1986 vaccine manufacturers were given product immunity. Under a direct discontinuance threat manufacturers began making protection demands rather than continue paying victim settlement costs or work on improving vaccine safety. Legislation passed that created a fund to pay off parents of dead or disabled children. The caveat would be any payments to parents or victims would only be made if either could prove their sudden demise was caused by vaccinations. Certainly both government and industry leaders knew that without a legal discovery process or knowledgeable physicians willing to testify most claims could easily be dismissed as coincidence rather than consequence.

Literally, at gun point, our vaccine industry dictated the agreement terms. They received total immunity and taxpayers would only pay for proven damages. The result was NCVIA. This act can now be viewed from a better perspective. Pharmaceutical company attorneys already aware of problems and growing liabilities confronting the tobacco industry completed what could be considered an ingenious solution for vaccine makers, but not necessarily for babies' safety.

Understanding NCVIA may help to get things into better perspective. Repeal of this fundamentally flawed law may even do more. If there were not known vaccine related injuries dating back to the mid-Twentieth Century, there would not have been a need for this law. With evidence certain serious childhood illnesses, such as, polio, were possibly preventable with vaccines created by Salk and Sabin, there could be no turning back. Vaccines were considered miracle preventive agents. Unfortunately, a lack of safety became evident when polio developed in a subset following Sabin's vaccine. After eighteen years it was finally removed from the market due to serious problems. It is entirely understandable why vaccine makers wanted product indemnity. They were aware some vaccines were potentially useless and more dangerous than any viral illnesses they were supposed to prevent. Getting this law into better perspective may be of help.

# 9

---

# The National Childhood Vaccine Injury Act

There was a growing problem related to vaccine safety. An agreement known as NCVIA would hold vaccine manufacturers and physicians harmless for any injuries caused by vaccines. Although NCVIA insinuated there would be injuries, no one seemed concerned about what might come to pass. No one could have envisioned vaccine makers would quickly begin rolling out more vaccines. Vaccine schedules would soon become crowded necessitating more shots during a single visit. Doctors that were responsible for ordering vaccines could not have had a clue about safety, because there was no need for individual or multiple vaccine safety testing. No one appeared to be concerned about how much mercury or aluminum would be injected into infants and children during a single office visit, or if they did, they did not fully understand the potential adverse consequences.

The Advisory Committee on Immunization Practices (ACIP) consisting of medical experts would have a final word on vaccine what and when. Newer vaccines, such as RotaShield and never before tried combinations, could be added without significant evidence of pre-marketing harmful effects. In the case of this vaccine there were warnings. Evidence RotaShield was not safe emerged relatively quickly with an increase in infants suffering bowel obstructions.

One morning in early 1999, I went to work at an inner city emergency department. My head nurse told me there was a vomiting baby in our pediatric exam room. A quick exam showed a toxic appearing, crying, dehydrated infant with a markedly distended abdomen without bowel sounds and blood in his diaper. X-rays showed an intussusception was causing the bowel obstruction. On admission the child's mother had reported her eight month old was up to date on all vaccinations. In 1998 ACIP had approved RotaShield to prevent viral diarrhea. Shortly thereafter, there were a growing number of similar bowel obstructions. I had no idea whether or not this infant's serious illness had been caused by this newly approved vaccine until I received word it had been taken off the market by ACIP. My job at the time was to get this infant to Children's hospital. I knew nothing about NCVIA. I trusted all vaccines were safe and effective. No one had asked whether or not this child had received the RotaShield.

Although NCVIA had additional important well known provisions, the emphasis was on keeping vaccines preventing childhood illnesses on the market. Although there was a provision requiring parents or caregivers receive a vaccine information disclosure statement, it was seldom done. A third and most important NCVIA provision was a process that would be necessary for reporting suspected adverse events. Manufacturers, without need to determine before marketing their products were effective and safe, would instead rely on reports about possible infant misadventures coming in from healthcare workers. Physicians, parents and caregivers, including third parties would become our vaccine industry's only safety net.

Without significant reports of possible harmful events assumptions could be made vaccines or combinations of vaccines, including their ingredients, were safe. Without major outbreaks among those vaccinated for mumps, measles, chickenpox, whooping cough, hemophilus influenza and polio, they could also assume vaccine effectiveness. Indirectly vaccine ingredients would get a free ride as long as adverse reports were few and far between. A poorly designed safety net utilizing a reporting system was and to this day remains fatally flawed. Safety has been totally contingent on a small number of adverse event reports rather than on the total numbers of adverse events.

RotaShield's package insert reported several cases of intussusceptions had occurred in a pre-approval infant study group. Having only five cases in infants given this vaccine, compared to one case in a placebo group was deemed acceptable proof that it was safe enough to become part of our first year vaccination schedule. It was not found safe. It is surprising this vaccine was removed from ACIP's vaccine schedule within one year. RotaShield may have already been under intense scrutiny. Possibly of interest, a physician member of ACIP had also invented a vaccine for the same rotavirus illness. Another possibility was ominous signs and symptoms of intussusceptions made a coincidental cover-up impossible. Remember ACIP knew the odds were high when approval was granted. Was ACIP waiting for vaccine failure before their next move? Did any babies die during those nine months it was allowed on our market? These are just a few questions about how much our vaccine experts actually knew, or better still, did not know about what they were doing.

Some might ask what members of ACIP were trying to prove. I am not pleased I did not know enough to complete a VAERS form. How many of my colleagues treated intussusceptions and never reported? There is probably no way of knowing, unless our insurance industry was keeping track. Allowing RotaShield on the market was a mistake. Immunity from liability became blemished in the aftermath. This example of a vaccine problem is pale in comparison with the much more sinister overall picture.

RotaShield's recall was an obvious example of how VAERS was supposed to work. RotaShield came and went almost without notice. Dr. Offit's vaccine was approved as one of two replacements by members of ACIP's committee. Subsequent surveillance studies primarily in Mexico and Brazil showed rotavirus vaccines have been associated with a lower number of intussusceptions, especially during the first week. In spite of evidence there continues to be a problem, the overall conclusion reached was the reduction in lost lives and hospitalizations significantly outweighed any vaccine risks. Unfortunately with an extremely porous safety net no one knows with certainty ACIP's assessment is correct.

As far as NCVIA provisions were concerned, it didn't matter because key players, physicians, were already on board our greater good vaccine train. There was no need to suspect a vaccine injury or file a report. If there was a problem it would, as in the case of RotaShield, soon become evident provided, of course, there was recognition of a correlation between a vaccine and subsequent illness. Appearances suggest physicians have fooled themselves and possibly deceived questioning parents and caregivers. NCVIA's subsequent reporting farce played into vaccine manufacturer's hands much better than expected. It only takes one pediatric vaccine expert proclaiming safety for all vaccines to convince thousands upon thousands of vaccine providers there is no problem. The only trouble might come from outspoken highly educated distrusting victimized parents and patients. Some parents may also be former trusting doctors.

Notwithstanding significant difficulty in proving cause effect, a major damage settlement was reached in 2008 with a doctor, who was able to show his daughter was permanently vaccine injured. As it turned out this was, perhaps, a perfect storm implicating a vaccine or its ingredients in an injury to a pediatrician's child. A vaccine or its ingredients had tinkered with and permanently damaged this child's cell mitochondria. In the aftermath of this poorly publicized settlement, if more doctors who believed their own children had been killed or damaged had risked coming forward, it is possible issues of coincidence would have long ago been replaced by consequence. Another possible reason why more physicians did not pay attention to this settlement may have been due to a rambling rebuttal published in the NEJM refuting any possibility this child had been injured by a vaccine. Dr. Paul Offit authored this refutation attempting to cast doubt on both this child's outcome and her father's motive. If more doctors had listened to parents of sick infants, instead of what they were reading or being told about safety and public good, there would have been many more consequence decisions.

Vaccine manufacturers, without adding any risk of liability and knowing what their DPT vaccine had already done, apparently had no problem adding adverse events to their growing list. Adding reports of SIDS and autism was, in my opinion, a simple defiant gesture. If no one, including physician parents, had an ability to come up with enough proof TDaP was a cause, it would be business as usual. And it was. NCVIA's key components designed to provide patients, parents and caregivers with information about what might go wrong, including what would need to be done were largely ignored. In other words, a vaccine information statement (VIS) necessary for obtaining informed consent and a VAERS submission in the case of an illness temporally following vaccination went largely unnoticed. Even if a mother was certain a vaccine had been responsible for her child's injury few doctors would dare offer her assistance. Fortunately, some brave physicians like Andrew Wakefield, listened to mothers and audaciously challenged Big Pharma.

It is extremely likely new serious adverse warnings are being added to a still incomplete list of vaccine events. Think for a moment how much more we know and still don't know today about our immune systems. Think also about, those horrendous revelations in the Vioxx drug case. Vioxx's manufacturer was aware their product could precipitate fatal heart events long before actual after marketing proof emerged. As many as 45,000 men and women were killed before there was need for disclosure. In the aftermath manufacturers paid fines and entered into insignificant settlements and went on with business as usual. Insiders who knew were silenced. If Vioxx death toll had not been as high pain relief experienced by the majority of users would have remained the greater good. How can vaccine manufacturers not be responsible for damages their products may cause when drug manufacturers can? Every parent of a SIDS victim or autistic child who received a DPT or TDaP should have legal rights to damages, in spite of NCVIA.

Similarly our vaccine industry has either known before or since the introduction of a vaccine there exists a far more sinister product side. What is currently known and published in vaccine package inserts should be sufficient for parents or caregivers to decide yes or no. Yes means a parent or caregiver has become informed and is willing to accept any inherently implied risks. A no decision will possibly set an unprecedented chain of events in motion. Scornful nurses, doctors, legislators and school systems will say no is unacceptable. Since when has no become an unacceptable answer? Nevertheless, in spite of informed consent no has already led to a mother's incarceration. No may lead to loss of public education, monetary fines, revocation of driver's licenses and inability to get future passports.

With protection afforded by NCVIA, Supreme Court decisions,

favorable media, lobbyist success and well funded pro-vaccine science research, our vaccine industry has become a new law of our land and master over babies' lives. What will come next? Is it possible our entire natural order has been changed? How can single events not be consequential and multiple similar events be coincidental? In cases of sudden infant death syndrome daycare workers have been sentenced to prison, because they could not prove they had not killed an infant in their care. When our AAP issues a statement SIDS should first be considered a result of intentional suffocation, the onus is shifted to a parent or caregiver who becomes guilty unless proven innocent. In cases of daycare deaths juries can be inclined to place blame on workers without evidence of any crime. Many parents of babies given a diagnosis of shaken baby syndrome (SBS) have been imprisoned based upon expert professional medical testimony. In these cases any possibility of coincidence was ignored.

I was once asked by a young U.S. Marine whether jostling within a carriage being pushed by a jogging parent could be a SBS cause. I whispered I wasn't an expert, but I suppose it was a possibility. That young Marine thanked me adding he had not shaken his child. He was going to prison. I later learned a fire retardant, antimony trioxide, commonly found in baby mattresses, carriages and strollers under certain circumstances, can be converted into a gas capable of killing or causing bleeding. I never thought to ask whether his baby had received a vaccine before dying. Once again, if I had known about intraventricular hemorrhage (IVH), noted in vaccinated ELBW infants, I might have been able to offer assistance. Vaccines should be treated like parents of SIDS and SBS babies, they should be guilty until proven innocent.

In order to more easily comply with VAERS, I proposed a change in an emergency department intake form. Ten years ago I recommended we ask the date of each child's last vaccination. Had this been agreed upon every sick child within thirty days of a vaccination could automatically become part of our VAERS system. This change would have possibly led us to confirming the fact we have been missing more than ninety-eight per cent of vaccine adverse events. Even a minor side effect, such as a fever or vomiting could be construed a harbinger of a more severe reaction the next time. If so, a medical exemption might be reasonable. No interest in my suggestion was apparent.

A recent Denmark study pointed out there was a seizure following the MMR in 1 of every 640 children. The first MMR given at one year of age resulted in 640 Danish children developing seizures. How valuable would an emergency department automatically submitted VAERS form become for seizures within 30 days of a vaccine? Extrapolating this Danish incidence to the United States would mean there should have been 5,700 VAERS submissions for first MMR related seizures alone. Our VAERS data base showed only ninety MMR related seizures or roughly 1.6% of what might have been expected. The 1.6% adds credibility to suspicions only 1-2% of all adverse events are being reported here in America. No reports means as many as 5,600 vaccine related seizures went unreported? This raises a question about how many of these children have gone on to become epileptic or have regressed into autism.

The failure of NCVIA created ostensibly to protect children from adverse vaccine consequences has not been coincidental. The primary objective was attained; namely, vaccine maker's protection. We have been left with a manufacturer's vaccine immunity act which must be repealed. No matter the consequence, vaccine makers must be held accountable for their product's safety and effectiveness. Without question study after study shows vaccines are neither safe nor effective, so allowing continued immunity makes no sense. In NCVIA's defense we can point out victims and families have received almost four billion dollars in compensation awards since 1986. A rebuttal might be over this same thirty years annualized damage awards have amounted to less than the total annual salary for a top vaccine maker's chief executive officer (CEO).

During this same period, an argument can be made a $30 billion a year liability free industry is flourishing in the face of unknown product damages. Looking at thirteen reported sudden infant deaths with diagnoses of seven SIDS among 13,500 TDaP recipients cannot be coincidence. SIDS deaths suggest correlation. Extrapolating this number to 3,000,000 TDaP recipients would equal 3,000 sudden infant deaths and who knows how many autism victims. If there was only one cardiac arrest in 13,500 recipients, extrapolation would equal 231 additional unexplained infant deaths. Defending this kind of data as nothing more than coincidental is ludicrous. Any vaccine apologist would need to know with absolute certainty mercury and aluminum could never be responsible for neurotoxicity and death.

How can parents, caregivers and doctors believe and trust grossly inadequate data and go on to defend this industry when statistical analysis clearly points to a correlation between vaccines and our current epidemics? Neither NCVIA nor Supreme Court decisions to help patch up liability loopholes will persevere in the face of advertising and medical study lies, or will it?

# 10

What about Coincidence
and Consequence?

In further testimony about coincidence absurdity something strange happened in Europe more than one hundred years ago. Thousands of infants mysteriously died during winter months for three consecutive years. Police concluded there were too many deaths to accuse parents of murder. Doctors had no explanation other than coincidence. Victims all under age of one year were being found face down on floors in homes of wealthy families rather than poor. Healthy crawling infants were suddenly dying. The cause of this mysterious winter epidemic of sudden unexplained infant deaths remained unidentified.

A famous Italian chemist, named Gosio, was asked to investigate. He quickly determined deaths were being caused by mildew generated, heavier than air, poison gas accumulating on floors. Smelling the garlic-like odor of arsenic's gas in the homes of infants who died was all he needed to settle on a killer. The gases origin was a fashionable pigment called Paris green found in wallpaper flowers made with arsenic. Wallpaper had become infested with mold in search of nitrogen found abundantly in this fabric's paste. During the winter months with heat, closed doors, windows and abundant moisture mold conditions were perfect. Mold consumption included both nitrogen and arsenic. Unwanted arsenic was expelled as a gas. Gosio hypothesized mold colonies were generating a poison gas. Unexplained infant deaths, in his opinion, were a consequence of Paris green being biovolitized by mildew.

The only solution for ending the epidemic would be complete removal of Paris green from homes and stopping further use of wallpaper and tapestries containing arsenic. This brought an end to sudden previously unexplained infant deaths and illnesses due to arsenic poisonings. Although the Lancet medical journal reported higher than normal arsenic levels were being found in sick patients who did not die, it took a chemist to determine a correlation. Deaths were a consequence of arsine gas exposure. Needless to say, William Morris adamantly defended his product's safety. Due to medical community resistance, Gosio would need to provide proof. Over unnecessary cruelty objections, he placed a rat in a large jar containing mold infested Paris green. Exposing an innocent rat offered those choosing to watch proof death would occur quickly. The exposure correlated with a cause-effect relationship. Arsenic's deadly gas was being created and released by a common household mildew. Is it possible similar events might befall those living better in an age of plastics?

Over manufacturer proclaimed innocence elimination of Paris green brought an end to what had been an epidemic of so-called coincidental deaths. Arsenic would still find its way into western civilization manufactured baby mattresses in the 1950's accompanied by antimony and phosphorus. A product designed to replace wool and cotton, polyvinyl chloride (PVC), was a chemically unstable polymerized plastic. It tended to de-polymerize. Stability and softness were attained by adding phosphorus. Arsenic was deliberately added due to a lingering belief it could kill mattress mildew. Due to PVC's highly flammable nature antimony was added as a fire retardant.

Phosphorus, arsenic and antimony have similar properties. They are in our Periodic Table's nitrogen group. Other than nitrogen each other element is a source for biological nerve gas weapons. Gases of all three elements have caused innumerable deaths in war time and in terrorist attacks. Is it possible PVC manufacturers did not know their new fabric was more than a cancer causing plastic and its ingredients might become deadly, if and when, mildew infested their crib mattresses? No proof of PVC safety other than fire retardancy was necessary. It was never tested for chemical ingredient safety on adults much less infants. PVC bassinets would begin appearing in NICU's and homes of those who could afford these new miracle products. Subsequent tests would show animal sensitivity with an increased incidence of skin rashes and asthma. Factory workers dying from cancer correlated with their PVC exposure. CNN's Dr. Sanjay Gupta reported a higher than expected rate of autism near PVC production sites.

There is a lot more to PVC's story. A Japanese manufacturer used methyl mercury to stabilize their PVC products. At process completion mercury was dumped into fishing waters of the village of Minimata, Japan. First signs there was a problem appeared when villagers reported seeing cats dance before dying. Soon infants, children and adults became ill with some deaths. A doctor working for the manufacturer concluded fish containing mercury was the cause. Cats fed mercury would have seizures before dying. Mercury had entered the aquatic food chain. Contaminated fish leftovers had been given to villagers' cats. Dr. Hosakawa was not allowed to speak out about his deadly experiments and business at Chisson's factory continued as a mysterious epidemic now with a known hidden cause was allowed to spread with support from the Japanese Medical Association. Eventually researchers identified mercury in victim's hair samples as far as five hundred miles away. A correlation was established and sick and dead family members became eligible for compensation. Company officials without disclosure stopped dumping, but it was already too late.

Finally villagers were joined by courageous scientists, defiant factory workers and student activists ultimately forcing the plant's shutdown. Post World War II Japanese government officials were forced to authorize payments for cleaning up more than thirty tons of methyl mercury. Victims received meager compensation for death or disability resulting from mercury poisonings. Had a cover-up succeeded there is no possible estimate of the extent of mercury induced human damage.

A closer look will show pharmaceutical and chemical manufacturing giants continue colluding and corrupting in order to prevent any bottom-line threatening process or movement from gaining momentum. It might be fair to say, both Big Chem and Big Pharma, with support from our medical profession, have risen far above legal containment with enough money and power to attempt mandating rescission of individual freedom of choice rights. Their continued success depends on doctors and legislators keeping their eyes closed and pretending not to see. Chemical companies such as Monsanto can practically do anything money can buy. Glyphosate also known as Round-Up is a carcinogenic poisonous pesticide following the deadly footprints left by DDT. Attempts to ban this pesticide in France are being thwarted by legislators under financial control of chemical industry lobbyists. Pharmaceutical companies are able to pay for the consequences of whatever they choose to manufacture, pay people who have the responsibility for approving, selling and enacting favorable legislation, or victims by simply adding these incremental expenses to their product price. Manufacturers of chemicals and drugs are liable for their product induced damages, if proof of injury is possible.

Amazingly pharmaceutical companies making vaccines are immune from product damages, with a fund to pay for injuries and, perhaps another one to eliminate opposition. Eliminating parental freedom of choice is an ethical and moral transgression of a basic human right. Asking doctors to carry out orders and remain silent must be construed a Nuremberg violation. The consequence of allowing a continuing vaccine SIDS autism cover-up will enable manufacturer's access to ongoing infant exploitation and experimentation without need for informed consent, provided healthcare workers continue to side with vaccine makers rather than infants and parents. More consequences of experimentation will follow. Can this practice with governmental sanction continue to be an acceptable norm? I say again as I did in 2010 no way.

Physicians and other healthcare workers must understand a gray area is appearing in medicine where consequences are overriding coincidences. Physicians must pay attention to any adverse event following a medication or vaccination. For example, failing to document a previously known penicillin allergy followed by a prescription for amoxicillin resulting in an anaphylactic reaction is considered a medical error or wrongdoing. A severe or possibly fatal consequence following will speak for itself. Physician liability will likely follow this adverse event. A breach of duty becomes a proximal cause for future settlement.

Similarly, a six month old child's mother reports her son became febrile after his first round of five shots at two months of age and then slept for 18 hours after his second round of similar vaccines at four months. This child's mother notices nothing is being documented and asks why. She is advised these events are not considered allergic. Without further comment a medical assistant prepares and gives five injections over an audible objection.

Case one fulfills malpractice requirements and a complaint may go to that doctor's professional liability carrier. In case two there are likely grounds for both malpractice and assault and battery. Doctor's indemnity protection offered by NCVIA will not prevail in court. Ignoring any possible prior adverse event is no different than failing to ask about penicillin. Failure to document a parent or caregiver's suspicion there was a previous adverse event, such as a rash or fever, is a medical mistake. Proceeding to give these same vaccines in spite of the risk makes for a much more significant problem. Attorney focus will be on the child's previously existing and more recent entries into their medical records. From my medical perspective both a failure to document, or documentation followed by automatic vaccine injections and a more severe reaction will speak for itself. NCVIA's physician indemnification will not likely be applicable in this situation. An attorney, who establishes a probable reason why this vaccine should not have been given, may be successful in prosecuting this case even if there appeared to be no immediate evidence of damage.

A better course of action would have been for the doctor to intervene followed by a medical exemption. Exempting this child from further injections is totally justifiable. Denying exemption and injecting a child, followed by any adverse event would equal proximal causation. Consequence would prevail over coincidence. Although, some may argue the greater good might be a factor, I do not believe a jury would rule in favor of a physician defendant. Callously ignoring prior adverse reactions may become a physician's worst nightmare. This scenario will likely play out, if vaccine mandates are allowed on a state by state basis. Once doctors, mid-level providers, nurses and medical assistants become aware of a greater liability risk for complying with mandates they may choose to do what is best for a child and themselves.

As this gray area becomes more defined, attorneys, depending on statutes of limitation, may start to subpoena medical records of dead and damaged children in order to establish time lines and determine whether there was a prior never reported vaccine adverse event correlating and causing a subsequent more severe event or death. Would it not be paradoxical, if attorneys viewing medical records of SIDS victims, for example, recognized a failure to report deaths that occurred within thirty days of their last vaccine? Is this a can of worms vaccine makers and physicians should fear? If NCVIA's reporting mandate, VAERS, was deliberately ignored by both physician and insurance third party, I believe, the worm is out and liability issues are real. Failure to report by either a physician or third party may not be sustained by a plea of ignorance. Both parties had a duty not likely alleviated by not knowing their responsibility under law. They either knew or should have known. Hopefully, in compliance with law, Pediatrix pediatricians submitted reports following each documented adverse event including those five deaths observed among the 13,936 infants inoculated in 356 NICU's during 2007-2012.

A nightmare of consequence predominating over coincidence will quickly become overwhelming when attorneys begin by asking defendants the meaning of VAERS. Not having knowledge of this reporting requirement won't be a good reason for failing to report any infant death or severe adverse event following vaccinations. No knowledge of VAERS will speak for itself. In looking to counter mandates, attorneys may become far more trustworthy for parents than doctors. Or better still physician fear that an attorney's discovery process will reveal a failure to document or report may override insurance company payments for performance compensation.

# 11

## Dancing Cats Silent Canaries 2010

*Dancing Cats Silent Canaries* was a story about my experiences, observations and evolving beliefs about what we have silently permitted to happen during my years in medicine. I chose to use dancing cats in my title to convey the neurological consequence of mercury poisoning. Dancing cats of Minimata, Japan symbolically represented another evolving cover-up orchestrated by a manufacturer. After silencing their own doctor cover-up help was needed from both the Japanese medical profession and government. Mercury poisoning can kill or create human behaviors resembling those seen in autistic children. Autistic children affectionately resemble dancing cats, possibly poisoned by environmental toxic metals, pesticides and the adjuvants in vaccines.

Silent canaries in a mine meant it may already be too late for mine workers. Singing canaries were an indicator air quality was acceptable. When canaries fell silent, it signaled either a poison gas was present or there was a lack of oxygen, or both. Miners would evacuate in order to survive, if it was not already too late. In my book silent canaries was a reference to the millions of babies who have suddenly died from what we have been told is natural rather than a consequence of some other factors. Victims of SIDS represent silent canaries, perhaps due to vaccines and possibly something associated with their crib environment.

*Dancing Cats Silent Canaries* linked SIDS and autism as being similar, but on opposite ends of a visible spectrum with several common denominators, including vaccines and mattresses made from PVC. Today, I believe vaccines, combinations and their adjuvant ingredients cause the majority of SIDS cases. Those children surviving vaccine exposures may develop neurological consequences including autism. It is as simple as it can be. Freeing our infant population from our current vaccine burden and their PVC surroundings will end these epidemics. This is a bold prediction. What greater harm could befall an infant with acquired maternal antibodies, healthy nutrition, availability of antibiotics, a supply of fresh water and chemically clean air?

With the half century mark close at hand for the American College of Emergency Physicians and my medical career, I can no longer be either an apologist for my profession, or vaccine industry funded CDC, FDA, HHS, medical science and legislative school alliances. On a daily basis I am finding it increasingly difficult standing by hearing the same old denials of danger. Then suddenly I heard a man say he would create a vaccine safety commission, if elected President. I saw there might still be hope, although I believed his chosen words might simply be an effort to gain voter support from a disenchanted vaccine concerned highly educated minority.

A few days after his inaugural address, perhaps, silenced by Big Pharma, nothing other than a few celebratory handshaking photos with some high ranking representatives of our chemical and pharmaceutical industries appeared suggesting everything was going as planned. Fulfilling a promise to a minority group of vaccine concerned mothers would no longer be necessary. King Pharma must have shown our President the vast amounts of money at stake, as well as, a potential for unlimited governmental liability. Coincidental deaths would not be allowed to stand in the way of progress. Perhaps, an ultimate slap in the face of concerned mothers was Dr. Andrew Wakefield's appearance at Trump's Inaugural Ball followed by a deafening silence. Soon there would be further defiant doctor and journalist coincidental deaths. Why had a trouble maker like Andrew Wakefield been invited? Was Trump acting naive or calculating?

A promised appointment of a rightfully skeptical Robert F. Kennedy Jr. to chair his so-called safety commission could not be allowed.

Business within the swamp would continue, perhaps, even murkier than before. Talk not walk had succeeded. Hopefuls, believing a mask on a $30 billion a year vaccine business would be stripped, instead became threatened by removal of all vaccine exemptions on a state by state basis. New cabinet physician appointees approved by King Pharma would carry vaccine industry banners. No one needed to pay any attention to dark side outcomes of premature vaccine baby studies. No one would need to know what might have happened to those babies, who had experienced NICU serious cardio-respiratory adverse events, after their next well baby visit for more injections. In spite of evidence there is the likelihood for a serious adverse event four times greater following five vaccines at once, there would be no warning or need to worry. Vaccines, poisonous adjuvants and toxic ingredients must be considered safe. Simply put, there is no choice other than compliance.

It has been said as much as things appear to change nothing really changes. As a physician, I can attest to this statement. However, in reality, most of what we were taught in medical school ten, twenty, thirty or more years ago is no longer true. Medicine without admitting change can deny the existence of new credible information one day and then embrace and take credit for it on the next. How will medicine be able to deal with today's premise aluminum can safely be injected into newborns tomorrow? On some occasions questionnaires rather than scientific studies are all that is required.

In *Dancing Cats Silent Canaries* I mentioned a questionnaire sent to New Zealand parents who had their babies die from SIDS. Answers to a question about what position did you find your baby, resulted in this country's 1989 campaign to stop allowing babies to sleep on their tummies. A seventy-four percent response suggested the prone position was a major risk factor. Without any need for a scientific controlled blinded study parent answers to a few questions resulted in a change for apparent good. There were thirty-three percent fewer crib deaths the following year. New Zealand's Health Ministry cautioned every one by suggesting it may be simply a coincidence. I wondered why there was no question asked about the date for their infant's last hep B, HiB, PCV or DPT, although I already knew there was no discernible need for this query, because any answers suggesting a correlation would not be explainable. A ninety percent or greater correlation with death within hours, days or weeks would need to be ignored. There were 2,800 unexplained infant deaths in the U.S. during 2015. How many had inoculations within the preceding thirty days and if they did had VAERS submissions?

By 1991 the United Kingdom instituted a similar back to sleep campaign with identical results. The U.K.'s Health Ministry used the possibility of pure coincidence. Perhaps, with the prospect coincidence was correct combined with no readily available scientific study, our AAP's president refused to allow an endorsement and there would be no recommendation for four more years at a likely annual cost of three-thousand crib deaths. Over his vehement objections, the academy ultimately adopted a similar back to sleep program. AAP's president went on to convey his opposing minority belief in a New England Journal of Medicine editorial. He predicted, in spite of contrary evidence on two separate continents, more babies would die from choking and aspiration due to gastro-esophageal reflux lying on their backs rather than their stomachs.

Thankfully, he was quickly proven wrong about more babies dying, but our current epidemic of infant reflux disease must in some way be related to something we are now doing that is new. I have no recollection any of my five children had reflux disease. Interestingly, those 239 infant ELBW NICU experiments reported increased reflux in both single and, more importantly, their multiple vaccine groups. We can agree infant immune systems reside within their gut. Tinkering with infant guts can and will lead to disaster. Reflux incidence in multi-vaccinated infants may be equivalent to earthquakes following fracking.

With no one in a leadership position willing to suggest there is any possibility of a relationship between vaccines, adjuvants and adverse effects, a subset of our infant population, remains at much higher risk. Unwelcome further research into any relationship between vaccines and a growing incidence of infant reflux disease will likely be stifled. Aren't SIDS and autism enough? Could our growing incidence of autoimmune diseases and allergies be further examples of unexpected coincidental outcomes? More likely they are being caused by accumulating adjuvants from more and more vaccines. Adjuvant fracking of infant's immune systems may be more consistent with resulting damage than tinkering,

In 1999 a scientific peer reviewed article appeared in Lancet about an unusual finding in guts of autistic children. The lead author was a pediatric gastroenterologist named Andrew Wakefield. His thirteen member research team at London's Royal Free Hospital with IRB approval had examined intestinal tracts of a very small number of autistic children with severe chronic abdominal pain. At that time United Kingdom's product manufacturer legal rights were in the process of a paradigm shift, so any suggestion a vaccine might be causing problems had to be unsettling. The onus for safety proof was being shifted from victims to product manufacturers. Suspected injured victims were being given the benefit of a doubt. Manufacturers would be required to prove their product was not causing a problem. The timing coincided with a growing concern about baby mattress safety. Evidence from a British chemist was suggesting older previously used PVC baby mattresses infested with mold might correlate with crib death. Meanwhile Wakefield's team was suggesting MMR vaccines may not be safe.

Reflecting for a moment on the possibility major mattress and vaccine makers would have to prove their products were not causing infant deaths or onsets of autism associated intestinal disorders must have overwhelmed respective petrochemical and pharmaceutical manufacturers, not to mention the Health Ministry and government. Britain's Health Ministry had already indemnified the same MMR vaccine makers whose products had already been withdrawn from the Canadian market. With two problems possibly looming, mattress poisoning issues would need investigation.

The Limerick Commission was established to dispel any notions a toxic mattress gas hypothesis was responsible for SIDS, also known as cot death. Several commission members, including a well respected pediatrician, proclaimed it would take less than six months to disprove a mildew PVC toxic theory. Dr. Barry Richardson, a chemist who had done the private research, was not invited to participate. Richardson likely knew more about mold and biovolitization than any person in England. Without Richardson Limerick's outcome would inevitably favor manufacturers. A pediatrician proclaimed chemists should stay out of medicine and stop scaring mothers. Richardson knew more about Gosio and mildew than any physician or chemist in England.

More than three years later the Limerick Commission concluded, in spite of reasonable evidence Richardson's hypothesis might be true, mattresses and mildew were safe, ending the controversy. It was too improbable so there was no longer any reason for parents to fear. Not unlike our 2003 IOM, the Limerick Commission concluded no further studies should be done. Meanwhile United Kingdom mattress manufacturers had time to conveniently remove and advertise their mattresses contained no antimony or arsenic. Limerick committee's pediatrician sent an editorial dutifully published in the New England Journal of Medicine claiming Health Ministry research had proven, once and for all, mildew and PVC were infant safe. As might be expected baby mattress concerns in England did not meet a need for consideration in America. In fact there was no need to even consider removing toxins contained in PVC. An additional fire retardant requirement would actually increased crib mattress antimony. Health Ministry attention could now be redirected toward Wakefield's 1999 comments and his published Lancet study.

I met with both chemists, Jim Sprott from New Zealand and Barry Richardson from England, on several occasions. I am almost certain I was the only doctor to have personal knowledge about their research and sincere belief a danger was present in older infant crib mattresses possibly explaining why a back to sleep campaign had been successful. I could not question their personal honesty and integrity. Choosing a path of least resistance was not in either one's character. Breakthroughs in chemistry and physics occur when an anomaly is encountered which leads to discoveries of paths never taken. Both of these men tried to advance our medical thinking, but were instead forced to deal with the consequences of their actions.

While the Limerick Commission deliberated, in conjunction with a local television station and Sheffield Children's Hospital, liver tissue samples were examined from Cot death victims and a matched group of infants who died for other reasons. Most members in both groups showed higher than expected antimony levels. Richardson's work had shown the gas of antimony, stibine, was being generated in PVC fabric by a common household mildew. Mildew isolated from two hundred cot death mattresses provided by parents were used in Richardson's laboratory experiments. Combinations of mattress PVC and mildew were generating antimony's poisonous gas. This finding had led Richardson to his toxic gas hypothesis. Liver tissue from infant cot death victims had the highest antimony concentrations. Richardson, not unlike Gosio, made his recommendation to remove antimony from crib mattresses and use new or used mattresses enclosed in a safe polyethylene plastic for each subsequent baby. Although average antimony levels in SIDS victims were higher, neither Britain's Health Ministry nor their medical community voiced any concern about how antimony had gotten into these infants' livers. No one seemed concerned a poisonous element added to PVC had mysteriously entered infants and was highest in cot death victims. Perhaps, everyone was more focused on another more threatening physician scientist named Wakefield. The Wakefield stakes were much higher. Barry Richardson's comprehensive scientific rebuttal was totally ignored.

# 12

## Wakefield and More

Research conducted by Dr. Andrew Wakefield during the late 1990's actually found abnormal intestinal lymph nodes in autistic children with severe gut issues not previously documented. Biopsies showed enlarged nodular changes caused by inflammation. Although not reported in Lancet, Wakefield's team had also uncovered more damaging evidence in these infants than his comment he did not believe the MMR vaccine was safe. He had found lymph node RNA sequences identical to those found in the measles component in the MMR. These infant immune systems appeared to have reacted abnormally.

Although abdominal pain was a symptom of wild measles, it usually disappeared with illness resolution. In this study children with a chronic disease may have become evidence of a MMR vaccine correlation leading to a major intestinal consequence. To Wakefield's credit he had educated himself on vaccine history. He knew more than anyone about both benefits and risks before making his 1999 statement that the MMR was not safe. Wakefield and Big pharma were on a collision course. Wakefield being right about a MMR danger was unacceptable to manufacturers, the British Health Ministry and mainstream medicine. Mothers concerned for their babies' lives could be silenced by successfully discrediting Wakefield.

During my career I had witnessed children with measles complaining of severe abdominal pain go to hospital operating rooms for surgical removal of their normal appendices. Wakefield's finding was more than likely an example of genetic tinkering gone astray. Ninety percent of this small group of autistic children had a new form of inflammatory bowel disease that must have frightened both manufacturers and Health Ministry officials. Rather than acknowledge a faulty vaccine had been inappropriately approved, attention was personally redirected toward Wakefield. Why bother with another commission?

In *Dancing Cats Silent Canaries* I went into detail about what happened as a consequence of Wakefield challenging the safety of the MMR vaccine. If his MMR fears were not containable, Wakefield would have to pay a dreadful price. Health Ministry leadership had already been compromised by money and providing MMR makers with indemnification. MMR products considered dangerous in Canada could safely be given to children in the U.K. Somehow new contradictory evidence in medicine, unlike other true sciences, is subject to unexpected resistance. Uncovering inconsistencies in parental histories, a slight deviation from IRB study approval or possible conflicts of interest might be a cleaner more definitive solution in dealing with Wakefield. No one needed to know more about a bad MMR vaccine as a plausible cause for what Wakefield's team had found.

As an example of medicine's willingness to compromise, resist change and reward poor leadership, there was a study commissioned forty or so years ago to prove there was no stomach bacteria associated with peptic ulcers. None of our FDA's carefully chosen eleven hundred studied samples revealed any bacteria putting to rest, once and supposedly for all time, the sixty year old hypothesis was false. Less than twenty years later two Australian physicians were awarded the Nobel Prize in medicine for identifying both an organism and a treatment. Their research confirmed a scientific article published in a late 1890's Polish medical journal. There was a business reason for trying to prove H. pylori did not exist; namely, gastric surgical procedures.

A more extreme side to the dangers of ill informed leadership had a direct effect on my personal life and the lives of more than fifty thousand American soldiers in Vietnam. All that really needed to be known about Indochina was contained in a book written by a French author who described in detail France's failure to understand the extent of reunification nationalism between north and south. Colonialism was coming to an end. Compounding France's mistake paranoid American leaders, under the guise of Communism fears and a manufactured Gulf of Tonkin incident, chose to jump into the abyss claiming it was for our greater good rather than the Vietnamese people, After two million people died defending their right to maintain freedom of choice American forces were defeated and fled the country. Vietnamese sacrifices led to their freedom from both Colonialism and Communism.

A valuable lesson for American leaders may have been lost in denial. There are many more examples of failed leadership in medicine, industry and government. Sadly, there seems to be no punishment for leaders who were wrong. Happily in the case of Vietnam resistance movements in America grew with mothers' marches soon joined by students, militants and returning Vietnam veterans. As an active duty officer and doctor I joined movements first in San Francisco, next in Jacksonville and finally on a march on Washington. Our resistance movement saved countless additional young American and Vietnamese lives suggesting any time there is oppression of human rights there will eventually be serious consequences. There will always be victims on both sides. Leaders of the oppressed will be most vulnerable to oppressor vengeance.

Robert F. Kennedy's 1968 presidential campaign promising an end to continuing carnage in Southeast Asia likely cost him his own life on a morning he claimed victory in California's presidential primary. Perhaps in response to his father's willingness to challenge the establishment Robert F. Kennedy Jr. has boldly taken a most difficult point position in the pro-choice vaccine movement. Kennedy like Wakefield and others has accused our vaccine industry, CDC and HHS of rampant collusion, corruption and a cover up. Offering a $100,000 reward to anyone able to produce an honest scientific paper proving there is no link between autism, mercury and vaccines has gone unpaid simply because none exist. RFK Jr., much like his father, has seen things as they are, and asked why? Why have we not reached the point of embracing an honest controlled scientific study between fully vaccinated and unvaccinated children? Why have we not embarked on a comprehensive safety study on primates before introducing known dangerous ingredients under the skin of our pregnant, newborns, children and soon to be teenagers. Politically sensitive and potentially important eyes and ears seeing the rising toll and hearing vaccine warnings are systematically being given advice to remain silent. Some are being forever silenced. I still believe it is not too late.

From my current prospective I see enlightened people are coming together in movements worldwide opposing our current establishment's position on unbridled use of a multitude of unsafe pesticides, genetically modified foods, vaccines, heavy metals, and chemicals. Contrary movements do not get media attention as a general rule. Anti-establishment organizations are considered rebels at best, trouble-makers or much worse. As their numbers increase media ignoring becomes impossible. Mothers against an ill advised Vietnam War and later drunk drivers eventually received much deserved media coverage and their marches and messages were seen and heard. Media journalists may have realized why they originally chose their profession. Street protests and local efforts to curtail pesticide spraying of toxic experimental genetically modified crops in school neighborhoods on Kauai, Hawaii have been legislatively thwarted at the highest chemical lobbied governmental level. At this moment resultant illnesses and defiant peoples' wills are of lesser value, at least until protest numbers reach a critical mass. Leaders opposing child safety from undisclosed poisonous pesticides must go. They will eventually be dismissed by defiant people. In the streets of Italy parents opposed to vaccine funded legislation increasing mandatory vaccines from eight to twelve for entry into school are openly marching and protesting. At the same time less corrupt government health officials in Japan, aware of the dangers posed by Gardasil, have caused a precautionary ban on its continued use in their country. Meanwhile, other countries, including America, well aware of Gardasil inflicted damages on young teen girls, continue to push for full compliance. Movements with common objectives tend to coalesce rapidly increasing their numbers and power. Ultimately corruption within governments and industries will become their Achilles heel.

Wakefield opened a vaccine inflicted wound. Those choosing to believe he had uncovered something important would need to be silenced. His situation would need containment, especially at a time when parents and lawyers were showing growing activist tendencies.

War would be declared on Wakefield by vaccine makers and for hire media spokespeople. Discrediting Wakefield would be accomplished by front page headlines proclaiming his Lancet study was fraudulent. Wakefield was ruthlessly attacked for his callous disregard for his study patients. In comparison, far more callous NICU ELBW vaccine studies had and would continue in America with a profound difference. In Dr. Wakefield's research there were no adverse events or deaths.

Wakefield remains an articulate thorn in King Pharma's side. He was a major participant in a banned in Tribeca movie *Vaxxed: From Cover-up to Catastrophe*. *Vaxxed* has been followed by a multitude of new revelations aired in well done documentaries and podcasts showing an extremely ugly vaccine under side. Wakefield was also behind a University of Pittsburgh study using vaccines and our vaccine schedule. Rather than use ELBW babies his study researchers used monkeys. Their entire monkey group given an infant's usual first year schedule of vaccines succumbed to neurological disabilities and death. Not surprisingly, well controlled and acceptable scientific journals refused to publish the results. Why would Wakefield choose to deliberately kill monkeys to make his point? Why would a chemist choose to sacrifice a rat to prove his point? Why would researchers repeatedly study adverse events associated with giving catch up shots to extremely low birth weight premature infants in their NICU's? Institutional Review Boards may have to think twice before approving any further vaccine studies on babies of any birth weight.

I still can't help but wonder what these same pediatric researchers would say if one of their own ELBW infants was scheduled to receive five vaccines at once. I could be wrong, but given this scenario, I would bet their answers would be, "No thank you." I cannot even imagine a NICU nurse or pediatrician becoming dismissive or hostile toward one of their own.

Richardson and Sprott were vilified as scaremongers. They are gone. Wakefield remains a fraud in the eyes of traditional medicine with no license to practice. Robert F. Kennedy Jr., who once was caught using drugs, remains an addict in spite of his noble efforts on behalf of children and our environment. In spite of once being convincing our President appears no longer concerned with vaccine safety. Nevertheless, our epidemics continue without signs of slowing as rebel movements increase in number and strength.

# 13

## From Where Did They Come?

My parents never knew about SIDS or autism. As a child I never heard of special education classes. During medical school no professors or textbooks made reference to young children mysteriously losing their ability to speak, who walked on their toes, flapped their hands, demonstrated repetitive obsessive compulsive behaviors and were more often than not antisocial. I was unaware of babies quietly dying in their cribs for no apparent reason.

During medical school l heard about an occasional crib death without explanation and a report about a few children who had developed unusual neuro-behaviors. Diagnoses of syndromes associated with sudden infant death and autistic symptoms were seldom seen. Following graduation and further medical training in the Navy during Vietnam, I helped to create a new practice of emergency medicine. Still no one was talking about possible drug or vaccine adverse events coming into emergency rooms. Medical journals devoted to emergency medicine made no mention vaccines might be a cause for pediatric fevers and seizures.

Several years into my emergency medicine career I experienced my first sudden infant death, but still no emergency room patients with autistic behaviors. The usual pediatric illnesses were chickenpox, mumps, measles, croup, whooping cough, unexplained fevers, diarrhea and on rare occasion a case of meningitis. These children all seemed to get better. I don't recall any deaths or subsequent neurological changes.

From the early 1980's to 2000 numbers of crib deaths, severe asthma attacks and infants with high fevers and seizures requiring testing for a source of sepsis inexplicably began to grow. One day I overheard a pediatrician explaining to the parents of a crib death victim that their baby had simply fallen asleep and had forgotten to awaken. I was astonished. Intuitively I knew better. All I really had to do was look around. New petrochemicals, pesticides and a growing number of vaccinations were emerging that I realized had never been tested for safety in rats, monkeys or humans before being introduced into an infant's environment. Soon after those revelations about the deadly consequences of DDT became known Monsanto and DuPont already had a pipeline of newer perhaps, more sinister products ready.

At a time when dangerous and deadly heavy metal mercury was being banned from topical disinfectants and gum soothing analgesics, it was still being injected into infants. I could not understand why mercury on infant skin was more dangerous than mercury under their skin. If NICU babies dying of Pink disease after being painted with mercury brought an end to this practice, how could anyone justify injecting similar age groups with mercury? In fact the injected vaccine preservative thimerosal not only contained mercury but also aluminum. Neither metal had ever been tested for safety. How could it? Thimerosal had been introduced five years before our FDA came into existence in 1939, which qualified it for a grandfather, no safety proof necessary, exclusion.

Although there were warnings from veterinary medicine this preservative was not safe for animals, it became a medically safe and acceptable vaccine component. There was a false belief mercury would be excreted and aluminum would effectively tinker favorably with our immune system response. Besides being considered safe thimerosal was cheap. Nothing further needs to be said about a lack of vaccine maker intelligence. At that point in my medical career I still appreciated Eli Lilly's graduation gift of a black medical bag. When a hospital on Cape Cod needed a sizable donation, I appreciated a gentleman named Lilly wrote a check. Nevertheless, I felt something was wrong.

By 1995 my SIDS curiosity had led me to New Zealand to explore a possible link to natural or man-made chemical environmental toxins.

New Zealand was thought to be a cleaner than average country, but it had the highest rate of SIDS in the world, especially among their native Maori populations. Unexplained deaths in New Zealand and elsewhere occurred more commonly during moist winter months. Intrigued further by a comment, which implied crib death did not occur without a crib had stimulated my interest. I set out to scientifically explore whether a newly developed crib mattress combining motion and sound might reduce New Zealand's death rate. There was data available which suggested baby rocking and communal holding reduced the risk. The same well known doctor proclaimed that in countries not using cribs, such as India, babies did not die from SIDS.

On my first New Zealand visit, I became aware of an Auckland chemist's hypothesis baby mattress polyvinyl chloride (PVC) interacting with mildew was causing SIDS. Mildew survived and flourished in the presence of nitrogen, moisture, warmth and darkness. Our Periodic Table of elements had three elements similar to nitrogen grouped together including phosphorous, antimony and arsenic. Mildew ingesting its major food source, nitrogen and releasing ammonia gas had the ability to consume and expel gases of nitrogen-like elements. If PVC fabric containing phosphorus, antimony and arsenic were ingested by this form of fungus, it was reasonable to believe their respective gases might also be released. A chemist's circumstantial evidence convinced me to abandon my research, because our innovative rocking mattress product contained PVC. I could not fathom what logic was used to justify adding three potentially toxic elements to an already dangerous product. What was wrong with wool and cotton mattresses that justified plastic replacements? Whoever was responsible probably never read about those infant arsenic poisonings in 1891-1894.

The chemist, James Sprott, advised me to go to London to meet with another British chemist, Barry Richardson, who had demonstrated a common household mildew found in PVC mattresses babies had died upon, could ingest one or all of these three elements and expel each as a potentially toxic gas. Following that trip to London I started thinking about chronicling my medical career with new evidence suggesting crib death had an environmental etiology. However, during a follow-up meeting with my New Zealand friend, I was advised to start looking at vaccines as another cause. I was certain these chemists were on to something of major importance. I knew backlash from the Health Ministries in New Zealand and the United Kingdom had profoundly affected Sprott's and Richardson's celebrated lives and careers. Any idea vaccines might also be causing more harm than good was personally discomforting. I became frightened. I put away my manuscript. I tried to forget about everything. I would not be successful.

Escaping my inner city emergency room had taken me back to Colorado's mountains not long after learning about a possible SIDS death in New York City only hours after a hep B vaccine was given. While doing a house call attending to an altitude sick patient, I watched a teenage boy wearing headphones, winding and unwinding a red ribbon around his index finger, relentlessly pace the hallway oblivious to my presence. My patient said, "His name is Philip and he's autistic." Unsettled by the sight of this 270 pound six foot seven giant, I composed a bit asking what she thought. "His DPT was the cause." Stephanie went on by saying her son was totally normal until the afternoon she took him to her Greenwich, Connecticut pediatrician for a well baby checkup. After receiving his boosters, Philip cried then fell into a deep sleep lasting more than eighteen hours. Unable to awaken Philip frantic calls were placed to her pediatrician who reassured her prolonged sleep was not unusual. Philip was in Aspen with his parents to attend a camp for autistic children run by the mother of Chris of similar age also on autism's spectrum. When Stephanie mentioned Chris' mother's name Sallie Bernard, I soon realized she had written a book comparing mercury poisoning signs with those seen in autism.

Several years later I sold my Colorado practice, but not before spending many hours with the mothers and fathers of Philip, Chris and others trying to understand more. Instinctively, I knew, if either of these vaccine injured children had died in their prolonged post-vaccination induced sleep, they would have been given the same SIDS diagnosis as that child in New York City. I left Colorado taking refuge in California choosing time in Monterey's Steinbeck country to work and put together a story about my journey, experiences and medical career observations. *Dancing Cats Silent Canaries* exposed my views on our epidemic of autistic children and victims of crib death, respectively. I pointed to an arguably strong link between SIDS and autism by suggesting similar toxic exposures during fetal development and an infant's first year of life could be either deadly or debilitating. Baby post-vaccine fevers in a PVC environment with mildew could be an even more treacherous combination.

At the time medical experts and fraudulent government funded studies were resoundingly denying any possible link between vaccines and the onset of autistic behavior. Nothing seemed to make any sense. And, after more than fifty years of research, SIDS remained a compilation of risk factors. These epidemics increasing in number in parallel with a growing list of vaccines suggested there had to be some correlation. Stephanie and Sallie had convinced me we were not being told the truth about vaccines.

When I originally returned from New Zealand in 1998, I had decided it was time to speak out about my growing concerns. A television interview was scheduled in San Diego. My interview about Richardson's hypothesis was balanced by airing an opposing view from the Chief Pathologist at Children's Hospital. His response was simple. He denied there was any possibility SIDS had a single cause and proceeded to call me a quack. Several days later in a personal meeting this same pathologist told me to my shock and horror, he believed parents and caregivers were more than likely responsible for SIDS. He went on to say there would be a new SIDS AAP policy. SIDS would be considered traumatic infanticide by suffocation until proven otherwise. My first question was how many autopsies he had performed on SIDS victims. He replied, "Too many." I next asked, "How many of those babies he had concluded were murdered." Mumbling somewhat his answer was none. Knowing his inconsistency, I indicated it was far more likely time will prove toxic crib mattresses and vaccines were the actual killers. He laughed as he stood up, stretched his suspenders signaling our brief meeting was over.

It didn't matter this man admitted he knew nothing about mildew or PVC. Somehow he knew vaccines were totally safe. At that meeting I mentioned the peak incidence of SIDS occurred during our vaccine schedule's first year. "Just a coincidence," was his immediate response. More than ever I was determined to learn more. Traditional medicine was obviously being run by a small subset of stubborn doctors unable or unwilling to acknowledge accumulating evidence of their potentially harmful policies and roles. A new AAP policy pointing a finger at parents, caregivers or daycare workers as primary suspects seemed more like a return to Salem for more Witch trials. Obviously, I had provoked a pediatric medical expert.

Medical experts had annoyed me for some time beginning in the aftermath of a harrowing emergency room shift. A police officer carried a seizing seven year old child into my trauma room. He reported her seizure had been continuous for more than twenty minutes. Sedation and intubation were successful and the seizures stopped. Subsequent testing revealed extraordinarily high levels of spinal fluid lead. The child's pediatrician concluded lead toxicity was not likely the cause for this child's epileptic seizure. He proclaimed there would be no need to lower her lead level using a chelating agent. He prescribed Phenobarbital to control her newly diagnosed epilepsy, in spite of lead laden paint found on a porch at her home. Medical experts were prepared to allow lead to remain in a young child's body and brain rather than consider using a relatively harmless life saving and life changing chelation product used previously on lead poisoned Philadelphia shipyard workers and more recently to remove excess iron from Thallassemia victims. I cannot understand why there has been a similar denial and failure to use chelation therapy in Flint, Michigan.

In the aftermath this same pediatrician asked me why I had performed a spinal tap and ordered an expensive test for lead. In my response I made reference to the fact that, if this child had died seizing would any pathologist have looked for lead as a cause or, if found would it have been just a coincidence? Ingested lead could not have been a cause. Years later I read about a sudden death of a police officer following a long day at a local indoor shooting range. Unusually fatigued he arrived home and went to sleep but never woke up. His death was attributed to acute lead poisoning. After my pediatric encounters, I was certain my chemist friends, Jim Sprott and Barry Richardson and the mothers of Philip and Chris possessed a much better understanding of these epidemics than any so-called experts denying there is a problem.

I was certain that New York City father, whose baby had died hours after being injected with hep B, also knew more than the vast majority of medical experts. He was responsible, in fact, for putting me in touch with an elderly retired pediatric doctor who advised me to take a look at our VAERS database. References supporting a danger were found. There were VAERS submissions for thirty-nine infant deaths following the hepatitis B vaccine between 1992 and 2002. One might ask how many infants were injured or died but were never reported? In the case of a hep B vaccine someone in authority, perhaps at ACIP, had decided it could be safely given on the day of birth, regardless of gestational age or birth weight, although no one could have possibly been certain whether this vaccine or it's ingredients mercury, aluminum, formaldehyde, or potassium, to name a few, might be dangerous for some newborns.

According to NCVIA our HHS and manufacturers were given primary responsibility for collecting and investigating reports of adverse events. This law mandated doctors initiate the process by providing feedback information whenever there was a suspected adverse vaccine event. Unfortunately, if an adverse event was not suspected, there would be no report. Or, if one was suspected and a report was filed, there would be no guarantee an investigation would follow. An additional more concerning possibility would be adverse events would be totally ignored by practitioners. I knew from my own experience a majority were being ignored and continued to go unreported. I was amazed to learn there had been MMR and DPT recalls due to reports of encephalitis, but there had been minimal publicity.

Medicine is frightened by iatrogenesis. Iatrogenic disease results from an activity of one or more persons acting as health professionals or promoting a service or product as beneficial to health, that does not support a goal of the person affected. It is an illness caused by a medicine or physician. Is it possible SIDS, autism, autoimmune diseases, Alzheimer's, parkinsonism, multiple sclerosis, amyotrophic lateral sclerosis and some cancers are examples of iatrogenesis? If not, what other answer offers a better more concise explanation for from where have these diseased come? Perhaps a look at our limited VAERS database will help.

# 14

## What about Our VAERS Database?

There were thirty-nine reports on file of babies dying hours, days or weeks after the hep B injection. Some might regard thirty-nine is an insignificant number when consideration is given to the fact millions of newborns were given this same vaccine from 1992-2002 and did not die. No one would likely argue this assertion might be correct, if thirty-nine represented one hundred percent rather than only one percent of all newborn post-hep B deaths. Upon taking a closer look at the VAERS demographics something else should have jumped off the page triggering an alarm. Approximately fifty percent of all reported deaths occurred in only two relatively small population states; namely, Oregon and New Hampshire.

One New Hampshire County alone accounted for three of the thirty-nine. These three newborns had been given a hep B shot containing identical lot numbers suggesting there had to be a direct link between this particular vaccine and subsequent death. Vaccines with identical lot numbers had been distributed in other states. How many other infants given this lot had died, but were never reported? Rather than raise a red flag warning certain vaccine lots might be more deadly than others, for inexplicable reasons, these deaths were in need of a non-vaccine related cause. Whether or not investigators had a suspicion nothing was apparently done. Meanwhile, sensing a problem, vaccine manufacturers moved quickly altering their distribution policy to avoid future similar lot death coincidence. After reviewing these deaths I began to suspect there had to be a well orchestrated ongoing cover-up. Three, possibly more of these deaths, were examples of iatrogenesis. Continued cover-up will inevitably lead to increasing numbers of vaccine catastrophes.

A too few deaths to worry about argument could still be construed as acceptable provided no one believed any newborn babies had encountered similar iatrogenic fates in our most populous states, but had never been reported. The daughter of the New York City father was not included. Eight years ago I suggested, based on physician surveys, less than one percent of doctors actually knew anything about NCVIA much less an existing VAERS safety net. For unknown reasons doctors, nurses and parents had received little or no educational materials. No queried physicians responsible for administering vaccines knew anything about this NCVIA requirement or another mandate that parents and caregivers be given a vaccine information statement (VIS).

In *Dancing Cats Silent Canaries* I revealed the possible seriousness of a failure to report hep B vaccine injuries. I thought more about that call. The father advised me his daughter's death had been attributed to SIDS, although initial autopsy evidence showed brain inflammation suggesting encephalitis. This diagnosis was nowhere to be found. I had advised the caller by definition SIDS could not have caused his daughter's death. As it turned out this gentleman was a powerful and influential man who would make himself into a hep B vaccine expert in order to testify before Congress. He warned our leaders about inherent hep B and other vaccine dangers using vaccine package inserts, his extensive research and Merck's manual. Apparently few congressmen were interested in listening to his cautionary rhetoric and nothing would happen. How many more infants would die? Was he considered just another quack? Was his expert testimony before a congressional hearing even considered by our IOM, AAP or ACIP?

Working in San Diego in late 2016, I learned of a similar story. A nine day old Wisconsin baby had died from apparent sepsis. Upon questioning her mother could not recall whether her baby had been given hep B, although I knew the odds were greater than ninety four percent. During 2016 this was the percentage of newborns that were given this vaccine in hospital nurseries. Sadly, more often than not without a word or parental informed consent this had become a customary near automatic practice. Manufacturer's serious adverse event warnings are not ever given. I urged this mother to find out more and, if a hep B was administered nine days prior to her baby's death, she should insist on a VAERS submission.

Both mother and grandmother became angry at my suggestion a vaccine may have been responsible for death. I informed both there was a law that required doctors to report events similar to those she had recently gone through. Before apologizing, I let her know that sepsis was listed as a cause of death in five cases during the 1992-2002 database time frames along with meningitis, encephalitis and pneumonia. I did not mention a most glaring and disturbing finding among those thirty-nine death certificates. Astonishingly, fourteen of these hospitalized sick babies were given SIDS as a final diagnosis. SIDS was apparently invoked as a hep B vaccine iatrogenic cover-up.

The CDC has attempted to explain a death following a vaccine was due to something already existing within an infant or child that was ultimately going to cause death or disability whether or not a vaccine preceded that inevitable outcome. In other words some infants are born with internal time bombs that will detonate no matter what. Vaccines were not triggers but innocently associated with being present when an explosion occurred. Although this barely fathomable explanation would eventually disappear from their website, I mention it only to convey our CDC's vaccine protective role. Vaccine blame can be covered by semantic suggestions similar to those Duke Researchers used to explain five ELBW deaths following multiple vaccines. Deaths would have occurred anyway. Iatrogenesis was not even a remote possibility.

It might be fair to conclude, these thirty-nine infants were likely the tip of an iceberg. However, with our vaccine industry in control, our FDA not doing its job, the CDC protecting and doctor experts proclaiming safety a continuing disaster seems inescapable. Could it be possible those thirty-nine represented only one percent of the total? If so, the real number of post-hep B deaths between 1992 and 2002 may have been well over fifteen hundred. Since 2002 the real number has to be much higher. Is it possible close to one hundred percent of SIDS victims have really been iatrogenic vaccine consequences? Is it possible, if Semmelweis was alive, he could ignore another obvious almost sacred pattern of denial?

Today, with no decline in SIDS prevalence combined with a further escalating incidence of Autism Spectrum Disorders (ASD) can there still be doubt fingers are, more than ever before, rightfully pointing to toxins in our environment, in hospital nurseries and physician offices. Infant death and disability in America already exceed all other civilized countries. Our AAP recommended schedule for newborns, infants and children contains twice as many vaccines as any other country. For some infants this schedule is a death sentence. With vaccine manufacturers free from product liability because of NCVIA and more recently by a Supreme Court ruling, it should not be surprising there is a world-wide push to increase vaccinations for all age groups, in spite of outbreaks of measles, mumps, whooping cough, chickenpox and shingles primarily among those fully vaccinated. At a time when safety is being questioned illness outbreaks provide direct evidence these products are also becoming less effective.

The time is long overdue to call a halt to the practice of continuing to mandate ineffective and unsafe vaccines before a significant percentage of another generation, in the name of money, is methodically destroyed. Those opposed to vaccines remain in a growing minority. Although our Supreme Court has given manufacturers free reign to continue producing ineffective and unsafe vaccines a minority justice's opinion has, once again, characterized vaccines as unavoidably unsafe. Did she hear that same testimony members of our IOM likely heard in 2003? Or, is it possible she knew about our CDC whistleblower pointing to a higher autism risk associated with giving a MMR to one year old Afro-Americans. She could have been referring to the MMR being unsafe for this subset. There can be no doubt our Supreme Court decision was fueled by overall fears about damaging the concept of societal greater good thereby exposing a huge industry and our American government to untold financial liability. What President Obama and our justices heard in private testimony was probably more troubling and ominous than what IOM members confronted ten years earlier.

Is it still possible with the balance shifting from safe and effective to unavoidably unsafe well meaning doctors caught in the middle no longer have a voice? If vaccine makers have no liability does any doctor harboring suspicion vaccines may be more harmful than good want continued immunity from liability for doing something inconsistent with their evolving beliefs? Immunity from one's own conscience is not possible. It is better to do nothing than continue to abide by old beliefs. Unavoidably unsafe is an oxymoron that must be replaced by avoidable and unsafe. Our VAERS database, our NICU experiences and vaccine manufacturer package insert warnings are enough for intelligent physicians to realize their own immunity may be sliding away for failing not to act responsibly.

Fifty percent of the VAERS reports in our hep B database came from several small states. Reporting sources were primarily third party insurance clerical administrators. Major insurance companies and third party administrators already have sufficient information in their databases that might prove vaccine iatrogenesis is not a cause for SIDS and autism. Another possibility would be, if their entities had been submitting reports our VAERS database might be overflowing. Without state by state court orders for discovery, would it not be wise for this industry to step up by adding what they may already know to our VAERS database? Deliberately withholding important information did not work for America's tobacco industry.

We know our insurance industry has information on vaccination dates and subsequent illnesses for every covered child. This assumption is correct if a physician's office billed the insurance company for a child's visit including charges associated with numbers and types of vaccines given and was subsequently paid. It is also reasonable to conclude these same insurance companies would have additional information on any office, urgent care or emergency room charges for any and all subsequent visits for illnesses of any kind this same patient may have experienced within thirty days following their previous visit for vaccinations. If these two assumptions are correct, it might be fair to conclude, our insurance industry is bound by law to report these associated illnesses or deaths as possibly vaccine related.

Going forward there is little likelihood insurance companies, including federally funded medical assistance programs, will begin to comply with NCVIA and VAERS or freely give up prior documentation citing cost as a reason. The insurance industry can afford to pay annually many hundreds of millions of dollars in top executive salaries, pay rewards to pediatrician vaccine compliance, increase premiums and decline payments, but cannot afford to abide by a mandatory law that was designed to protect children from vaccine injuries. Outrageous would best categorize insurance companies deliberately withholding VAERS related information.

It is possible insurance companies have vital information in their database that could vindicate our vaccine makers. Data showing few childhood deaths occurred within thirty days of a vaccine office visit might go a long way toward quieting and slowing a growing pro-choice movement. Another, perhaps less desirable outcome, would be the opposite more deaths and neurological regressions than can rationally be explained by internal time bombs. Ultimately, American insurance companies must do what is morally right and in the interest of health. Insurance companies must be held legally accountable one way or another.

# 15

---

# Backlash

*Dancing Cats Silent Canaries* predicted there would be major backlash if oppression against vaccine resistors continued. It has grown. There has been an extremely well orchestrated intensification on all levels likely fueled by corporate power, greed and money. Pharmaceutical heavily funded lobbyists have strengthened their hold at both the federal and state level. Attempts to subpoena whistleblowers within our CDC, who possess vaccine damaging evidence, are being suppressed. At a time when an indicted author of a fraudulent Danish study allegedly showing no link between mercury, vaccines and autism is being allowed to run free and states are attempting forced vaccine mandates on free citizens something is seriously wrong. Is it possible a decision was made to deliberately keep citizens, especially American parents and physicians, in the dark? Keeping whistleblowers quiet and allowing an international thief his freedom is, in my opinion, an unacceptable turn of events.

Currently any attempt to do a controlled scientific study comparing the health of unvaccinated and vaccinated is being stone-walled by so-called professionals in fear of the outcome. Any attempts being made to try to identify infants perhaps more vulnerable to certain vaccine contents are being stymied. The good news is coincidental death whenever a baby dies following an injection is a term gradually being eroded. In some cases consequence has replaced coincidence.

The legal expression res ipse loquitor, which means a thing speaks for itself, has been used to justify damage awards, if there is no more plausible explanation. Any death or symptom of possible neurological disease regardless of patient age that occurs within hours, days or weeks of a vaccine should be allowed to speak and be heard above mandate clamor professing vaccines represent a greater good. This specious argument is no longer morally valid. Philosophically speaking no good can come from an evil. Vaccines, vaccine combination, adjuvants, such as, aluminum and mercury, other ingredients and contaminants are too evil to trust another day.

The internet has given parents and caregivers an exponential learning opportunity. Truth is being revealed in documentaries about ineffectiveness and avoidable dangers inherent in vaccines, ingredients and numbers. A majority of doctors continue to carry safe and effective banners with an occasional internal dissenter daring to violate or question the doctors' code of silence. One pediatrician with unvaccinated, partially vaccinated and fully vaccinated children in his practice is trying to submit a paper with his own evidence. He is being ignored. He can show evidence that his unvaccinated children are much healthier with fewer office illness visits. This group of more than five hundred children has only one autistic child. A complete opposite is evident in his fully vaccinated group. These children are more prone to illness related office visits with fifteen on autism's spectrum. A middle partially vaccinated group is slightly more healthy than his fully vaccinated, but still has six with autism. An honest conclusion might be an extrapolation of his practice experience makes an excellent argument to delay or not to vaccinate.

A study in Mississippi confirmed this state has the unhealthiest children in America. A plausible explanation might be data which shows a near perfect ninety-ninety percent vaccine uptake. Only one in every two hundred children is not being kept up to date. Mississippi's infant death incidence is twenty five percent higher than our 6.1 per 1000 live births national average. Parents in this state, based upon data speaking for itself, may need to say no more vaccines until manufactures and medical experts agree to prove they are not responsible. Manufacturers should be forced to agree, or better still, take their products off the market until safety is proven. This is clear evidence something is terribly wrong with what is being done to our children. A closer look at Georgia and Arkansas will show similar infant death rates and illnesses. Is it possible government funded health plans and free vaccines for our medically indigent practically guarantee there will be serious adverse consequences? Who will ultimately pay for soon to be explainable vaccine related outcomes? Special education classes for our vaccine injured cost tax payers in excess of one trillion dollars last year. Can there be any doubt our insurance industry has much more vaccine incriminating evidence they cannot afford to make known. If this can be substantiated, there will be unprecedented backlash. Why should our health insurers pay for damages caused by vaccine makers, federal agencies and health care providers?

I heard a doctor telling a questioning parent the HPV cancer preventing vaccine Gardasil, based upon a placebo controlled study, would be safe for her daughter. This child's mother asked whether aluminum hydroxide was safe. The doctor immediately said, "Yes of course." She next asked what placebo was used to compare side effects of aluminum containing Gardasil. The doctor responded, "A placebo is usually saline or sugar." A social media informed mother told the doctor the control placebo group had been injected with aluminum hydroxide. Not surprisingly when both groups were compared the desired outcome had been achieved. Not unexpectedly reported side effects of Gardasil with aluminum and placebo with aluminum were similar.

This terribly flawed safety study should never have qualified as scientific, although there have been far worse so-called vaccine studies. Imagine testing a vaccine on a dying patient and conclude the vaccine was safe because the patients died. In this case someone must insist on asking about the health of both Gardasil and placebo groups at three, six, twelve and twenty four months post-study rather than three days. Whether this particular doctor learned more from a parent than his Gardasil manufacturer doesn't really matter. Our real problem is school systems, particularly teachers and school nurses know much less than the mother or doctor. Nevertheless, teachers and nurses are being forced to exert pressure on uninformed or deliberately misled young girls and boys. California law allows for Gardasil to be given without parental knowledge much less consent. What chance does an emergency physician have dealing with a vomiting teenage girl without a reliable history, especially if this vaccine was given secretively unbeknownst to her parents. A Canadian study reported ten percent of young girls injected with the HPV vaccine end up in an emergency room within thirty days. How can anyone conclude this vaccine is so safe for young girls similarly aged boys should also be given the same? Boys seem to already be at higher risk for adverse events.

I recently saw a fifteen year girl with a diagnosis of Postural Orthostatic Tachycardia Syndrome (PoTS) with a dozen emergency room visits during a twelve months period. She had been given Gardasil. Her father had never been advised by his daughter's doctors that PoTS was a documented serious heart related Gardasil adverse event. My first instinct was her doctor specialist didn't know, but how could this be possible? My second thought was her doctor chose not to tell. Regardless, necessary documentation is already present in her insurance company's never reported database. It will only be a matter of time before someone subpoena's her medical records and finds the correlation.

Teenage girls are collapsing in doctors' offices immediately following this injection and some have consequently died while others are becoming disabled for life without legitimate proof this vaccine can be of any cancer preventing benefit. Gardasil related suicides are increasing. While Gardasil is being denied licensing rights in other countries, because of known consequential adverse effects, it remains on our market. In spite of the fact manufacturers admit it has not been proven safe for female reproductive organs the marketing effort is intensifying. Testing on animals to determine infertility outcomes was not deemed necessary before rushing into this most lucrative market. There is little doubt many vaccinated teenage girls will never have babies, but may still get cervical cancer. Few individuals in authoritative healthcare positions are paying attention to either short or long term consequences of Gardasil or Cervarix. Primary Ovarian Failure (POF) is, not surprisingly, on the increase.

There is an old saying, if a tree falls in the forest does it make a noise, if no one is there to hear it hit ground? Likewise if infants and young children are falling victim to toxins and vaccines do they make any noise, if no doctor, nurse, insurance company or parent dares to hear and report? There are growing numbers of young once vibrant teenagers whose lives have been destroyed after receiving one of the three recommended vaccine doses. If only hospitalizations for nausea and intractable vomiting following a first Gardasil injection were being tracked by our sophisticated insurance industry and legal system this product would be forced off our market. If a hospitalization occurred after a single dose shouldn't conscientious doctors be allowed to provide a medical exemption from dose two and three? Should a parent be notified by their insurance carrier a possible vaccine related hospitalization or emergency department visit occurred in order to comply with existing law?

Whenever there is an adverse event after a first time injection of any vaccine should a doctor or mid-level provider become liable for any consequences of a second or third injection? In my medical opinion a mandatory medical exemption should become a new standard of medical care following any adverse event no matter how mild. Deviating by denying a possible prior cause effect should become an act of malfeasance. If damage of any kind follows deviation by further injections, there will be grounds for malpractice

Dr. Diane Harper, who designed phase two and three trials for Merck's Gardasil, is very cautious. In a 2009 CBS interview with Sharyl Attkisson she cautioned parents about both risks and benefits clearly stating maximum effectiveness may not be greater than five years. In the meantime Merck says there is no increased incidence of sudden death, non-Hodgkin's lymphomas, suicides or ALS, also known as Lou Gehrig's disease following their vaccine, although the company admits VAERS investigations continue. Another doctor on Attkisson's report clearly stated he was absolutely certain his daughter would have been better off with cervical cancer than the adverse events following this vaccine. I no longer have any doubt insurance companies are holding the pin on this vaccine grenade. The eventual backlash is already becoming palpable.

It goes without question nothing will be reported in newspapers or on television without editorial approval. Attkisson's report about Gardasil was an obvious exception. Nevertheless a journalist in Boston was cleared by her editors to recommend vaccine objectors should be hung by the neck until dead. Does this apply to that same doctor who said no to Gardasil for his other younger not yet damaged daughters?

Over vehement backlash to both content and tone Boston Herald's editorial board declined to make a retraction. Being from Boston I was embarrassed by classic media based bullying borne from ignorance. Reader backlash had to be ignored.

Possible parental refusals when the truth about higher autism risk for Afro-American children when given the MMR vaccine at age twelve rather than twenty four months might result in this journalist and editor thinking twice before issuing a similar distasteful comment. As it stands a CDC scientist has already provided evidence concerning this hard-to-believe deception. It is doubtful when Afro-American mothers and caregivers become aware their one year old is at higher risk of autism, as a consequence of complying with our vaccine schedule, they will not become resistant. Will they be denied healthcare and public school? Civil rights legislation reinforced religious rights making mandatory vaccines a civil liberties violation.

Any backlash for resistance by Mississippi mothers would likely be termed criminal. Once again, what would those Boston Herald editors recommend as a punishment? Every doctor or mid-level provider should know about this study, regardless of whether or not a whistle-blowing high level CDC scientist is allowed to go public with his evidence that a vaccine link exists between MMR and autism in a likely more vulnerable subgroup. Any admission might also lend credibility to high autism incidence among Minnesota MMR vaccinated Somali Americans.

Night time network comedians have chosen to verbally abuse any person hesitating or objecting to vaccines. Programs seldom allow any scientific rebuttal. On one occasion NBC's Today Show gave Dr. Andrew Wakefield an opportunity to defend his belief the MMR was dangerous, but not without counter balancing his words with their own medical expert's contrary accusations. Dr. Paul Offit's vitriol included derogatory never proven accusations of fraud. On another occasion Robert F. Kennedy appeared on Fox. The host was fair and seemed to agree with Kennedy's premise we are destroying a generation of children with mercury, aluminum and vaccines. Although short in time Kennedy's interview was a positive step in the direction of pro-choice. Parents and caregivers rallying behind informed consent cannot be condemned and hung for saying no. Honest media journalists will ultimately report the truth about vaccines, whether they currently know it or not.

In Italy thousands of people have demonstrated in the streets against having their children banned from public school and fined for vaccine non-compliance. Their backlash is against a legislative proposal for a thirty three per cent increase in mandated vaccines. Italian news stations show demonstrators, but at the same time, carry stories of a giant pharmaceutical vaccine manufacturing company's plan to build a new billion dollar plant on Italian soil. New jobs are more important than vaccine damages one might conclude. Has anything really changed since Minimata? Who can parents trust? By now most would agree that anyone with a financial interest promoting potentially dangerous products should be avoided.

Doctors who pretend vaccines are both effective and safe must be confronted with facts. They have no scientific proof any vaccine, combination of vaccines or their various ingredients are safe. Any doctor who tells a pregnant woman to get an influenza shot, more often than not containing mercury, does not know this shot is less than effective and is associated with a twofold or greater risk of a spontaneous abortion. During America's HINI flu epidemic spontaneous abortions among women given the vaccine increased more than seven-fold. Vaccine promoting doctors with a financial interest cannot be trusted.

Medical organizations, it could be argued, have a duty to speak out if there is evidence of a vaccine danger. Based upon my history with ACEP, I proposed there be an endorsement of NCVIA, VAERS and VIS. Establishing an urgently needed educational program for emergency physicians had to become a highest priority. To date I have asked many well known emergency physicians the meaning of VAERS with no correct answers. No one knew anything about our vaccine adverse event reporting system. Next, I proposed each electronic medical record (EMR) contain a triage question about every patient's last vaccination date (LVD). This could become a proactive means for determining if a vaccine had temporally preceded an illness, such as, vomiting, fever, seizure, encephalitis, sepsis or death. Sadly there was very little interest in either of my suggestions.

My suspicion is there are serious adverse vaccine events being missed on a daily basis in each of more than five thousand ED's across our country is likely correct. Total annual vaccine related illness misses could easily exceed one million. Perhaps one million children becoming ill enough to show up in an ED only to be given, in spite of vaccine insert warnings, a diagnosis unrelated to recent vaccinations. At the very least every child having a febrile seizure within four weeks of a vaccine known to cause convulsions should have an injury timeline. A subsequent disability might make them eligible for compensation.

No one I have spoken to in an organization I had helped create believed adding a simple suspected adverse event report could strengthen our vaccine safety net. One colleague sensing my passion brought up this topic at an AMA meeting and was resoundingly booed back into his seat. Another colleague simply said too much work. Most medical organizations cannot be trusted because they rely on income from companies manufacturing drugs and vaccines. On vaccine issues no one at our AMA wants to go there, possibly reminiscent of another tobacco era.

Our current news media, including newspapers and television stations, as alluded to earlier, have fiduciary responsibilities to their corporate owners and advertisers. During my investigation into the SIDS death hypothesis, I was advised a CBS 60 Minute team led by Ed Bradley had gone to the United Kingdom to conduct interviews with the chemists responsible for suggesting there was a crib mattress danger. After viewing their documentary, editors shelved and refused to air their program. According to a retired journalist, CBS network affiliates were advised to remain silent. When one considers America's news media is now largely controlled by King Pharma and our petrochemical industries this should not be surprising. At this moment no media personalities can be trusted, but there will be a change. Journalists' backlash to being muzzled will begin happening when important well researched stories are shot down without good reason.

Backlash will intensify as evidence of wrongdoing inevitably continues to appear. Doctors cannot staunchly and arrogantly defend vaccines without being forced to conclude injections of neuro-toxic aluminum on days one, sixty, and one hundred and twenty pose no problem for infant's cardio-respiratory, gastrointestinal, neurological or immune systems. Bias created by insurance company vaccination rewards based upon available evidence of risk exceeding benefit cannot be construed as either ethical or moral. Autoimmune diseases created by the adjuvant aluminum will become more apparent. Follow-up long term outcome studies by ELBW baby researchers would in all likelihood reveal long term benefits or risks of bringing these infants up to date. In my medical opinion, such a study would expose an ugly downside with barely imaginable consequences.

# 16

Babies' Lives Matter

Truth about overwhelming risks associated with vaccines, vaccine combinations, adjuvants and other ingredients already exists. Manufacturers and researchers have acknowledged a myriad of serious adverse events, including deaths in immediate days following vaccinations. No one has any right to make an assumption these events do not continue with each forthcoming vaccine round. No one has any right to assume every infant and child can tolerate the total amounts of first year aluminum. Everyone has a different "tipping point." Sudden unexplained childhood deaths, regressions into autism and immune disorders attest to injuries sustained in early vaccine rounds. One more vaccine could be a final tipping point. Even with a 1.6% sample of what can go wrong vaccines are obviously causing more havoc and harm than good. With just a glance at available evidence everyone should be able to conclude reasons why thirty two countries have lower infant death rates and American children are among our planet earths unhealthiest.

Federal agencies such as the CDC, FDA and HHS have a duty to protect babies' lives. None appear to be doing so. None can be trusted. Rampant current evidence of corruption within and between these agencies and vaccine manufacturers intensifies a louder cry for no more. Perhaps, these agencies find themselves between a rock and a hard place. Simply put, the truth will devastate a current $30 billion dollar vaccine industry. In the process there will be revelations senior scientists and executives were flagrant liars trying to protect their jobs rather than babies' lives. Fearful parents must be the ones coming forward to rescue infants from corporations and agencies out of control. More than ever parents must choose to listen to an emerging group of wise humanitarian doctors who have placed their lives on the line.

Dr. Andrew Wakefield, for one, had no knowledge about the extent of serious adverse events parents began to attribute to the MMR. There is no reason not to believe he began listening to mothers. Wakefield's life forever changed the moment a mother of an autistic child, who was suffering from intractable abdominal pain, told him she intended to kill her child before committing suicide. Admitting he knew very little about autism his prior research into Crohn's disease, an intestinal autoimmune illness, may have convinced him something needed to be done, not knowing there would be serious almost unimaginable consequences stemming from his decision. A subsequent IRB approved peer reviewed paper was published by Lancet. During a press conference his response to a question about MMR's safety set a wave in motion. Wakefield believing babies' lives mattered unknowingly placed his medical career in jeopardy.

The Health Ministry and media with pharmaceutical industry financial support ultimately took Dr. Wakefield down, forced Lancet to retract his published research and discredited any link between MMR, gut disease and autism. It was not easy. In 2006 King Pharma underwrote a powerful media covered front page warning to Wakefield and other legitimate dissenting researchers at the same time they were funding research on NICU held ELBW infants. Wakefield had no reason to believe he had not been honest in complying with his IRB. A London Sunday newspaper with strong ties to a vaccine maker chose to publish a new version of his research. Clamoring Wakefield was medically unfit to retain his license a vaccine journalist attempted to destroy both his career and life.

Amazingly, it would take more than three years of testimony before the remaining members of Wakefield's research team, who had refused to recant their findings, were stripped of their medical licenses. I believe any conclusions Wakefield was guilty of callous disregard for babies' lives were totally unjust. Wakefield's lead researcher would later be vindicated by a judge who literally described his original trial as a kangaroo court. Later research would confirm his team's findings. A University of Pittsburgh animal study, noted earlier, using our recommended first year vaccine schedule on monkeys resulted in one hundred percent sustaining disability or death. There were no major scientific publications willing to publish these findings. A study demonstrating the devastating vaccine adverse events on monkeys was scientifically unacceptable. How was this possible, when studies on ELBW infants showing significant adverse cardio-respiratory events, strokes and possible deaths, after peer review, were published in pharmaceutical supported medical journals? Most disturbingly our NICU authors, looking at their own data, concluded there needed to be more ELBW research. How many infant experiments will be necessary before they learn what parents already know? Can either doctors or parents afford to trust published peer reviewed science? Should parents trust a doctor who tried to help save babies lives costing his career?

Whenever anyone questions societal good, discussions must shift to actual benefits posed by a growing list of vaccines, primitively created in a variety of ways, sometimes in distant countries. We are being told without MMR vaccinations thousands will die from measles outbreaks. Rather than defend a suspicious MMR vaccine history, we are being scared by CDC reports there were twenty one thousand cases of measles in Europe with eighty six deaths last year. Problems are falsely being attributed to individuals never vaccinated who are being allowed to travel spreading disease to places like America. Medical experts warn us unless ninety-five percent of people are vaccinated these epidemics will grow killing vast numbers of innocent victims without mentioning vaccinated individuals appear to be at high risk.

What is not being reported is the risk of death from any illness, such as influenza, is more associated with a need for hospitalization than a virus. Hospitals and hospital employees are MRSA reservoirs making hospitalization a major risk for iatrogenic infections.

# 17

Warnings from the Past

Many years ago Dr. Arnold Relman, the New England Journal of Medicine (NEJM) editor, warned the medical profession about growing dangers inherent in a pharmaceutical takeover of his beloved journal and eventually our medical profession. Largely ignored he ultimately resigned when drug advertisements took over his journal's first twenty pages. Twenty years later, his successor, Dr. Marcia Angell, upon her own retirement, seemed to reinforce her predecessor's warnings by saying she could not be certain any articles published during her tenure were scientifically trustworthy. An example she may have been alluding to may have been our CDC's now infamous Danish study alleging no link between the MMR, mercury and autism. After NEJM's publication New York Times editors proclaimed this peer reviewed paper proved, beyond any doubt, vaccines, especially MMR, were safe.

Although this research was later shown to be statistically invalid and scientifically fraudulent several media medical experts, including Paul Offit, remained adamant this study was valid. Prestigious NEJM editors never retracted this study or admitted its primary author had been indicted in Denmark for money laundering embezzlement and fraud all at our CDC's expense. I am certain letters directed to Dr. Angell for editorial rebuttal went unanswered and ignored. As it turns out contents of most published scientific articles are carefully filtered by a single source capable of excluding non-compliant, but not necessarily fraudulent, science. New York Times editors also felt there wasn't any need for a retraction.

Delays in releasing truth can result in the accumulation of billions of dollars in profits. Pharmaceutical profits can be used to pay out millions in future fines. Without any worry about consequential payments for childhood damages thanks to our NCVIA vaccine makers can go about business as usual. Vaccine taxes to fund proven injury compensation can be increased should billions in current reserves become exhausted. Can doctors really trust pharmaceutical inspired literature being dumped into medical journals? How long will it take before more doctors look around and see what Relman saw happening in the 1980's and decide to no longer listen to our CDC's propaganda?

If parents and caregivers cannot afford to trust pro-vaccine doctors and scientific journals, can they afford to trust vaccine manufacturers? As crazy as this may seem my answer is probably yes with a degree of caution. Vaccine manufacturers provide information about known and post-marketing reported serious adverse events in their package inserts. A list of vaccine ingredients and lot numbers can also be found. The doctrine of informed consent currently being upheld by our AMA is a patient right. It is testimony a patient, parent, or caregiver knows about vaccine benefits, risks and alternatives. If a TDaP insert, for example, includes SIDS and autism, informed consent means a recipient accepts these risks in return for an implied protection against catching diphtheria, tetanus or pertussis. There is no recourse, if at some future time an allegedly protected person catches one of these illnesses. Parents need to be told there is no implied guarantee a vaccine will remain effective. They should also know an alternative treatment for pertussis is an antibiotic known as Zithromycin.

If recipients go along without reading about or being advised of possible risks, there can be no informed consent. Vaccine administration without informed consent can be construed as assault and battery. Nurses, mid-level providers and doctors, who fail to obtain written consent prior to administration, can be found guilty. Healthcare organizations requiring employee vaccinations without obtaining informed consent may find themselves on extremely thin legal ice, if firing is their alternative.

Notwithstanding maker admissions of possible vaccine adversity an informed mother, who refused to allow vaccination for her son, recently spent seven days in jail. Overriding her failure to give informed consent was a greater good concern. When a judge can incarcerate an informed non-consenting mother by denying her freedom of choice our Constitution is being overwritten. If ultimate arguments are based upon a now debunked notion of herd immunity, problems caused by vaccines are of greater individual concern. Theoretically an unvaccinated child with measles should never be able to infect a child vaccinated against measles, unless an original vaccine series was ineffective.

Lessons from our past can but should not be ignored. King Pharma is nothing more than another, perhaps smarter and more dangerous version of Big tobacco. Big tobacco paid hundreds of billions of dollars for damages in order to be allowed to stay in business, while King Pharma's vaccine maker damages are being paid by recipients, insurance companies and taxpayers. Keeping vaccine makers with their current suspect products in business by paying for damages no longer makes any sense. If manufacturers trusted their products, there would never have been an indemnification need.

Serious vaccine warnings from the past can be traced back three hundred years. Dangers associated with Paris green infant arsenic poisoning deaths go back one hundred and thirty years. Deaths attributable to asbestos have been found in Marco Polo's writings. Individuals who have been willing to speak out against conventional thinking have made a difference. Rachel Carson helped get rid of DDT. Semmelweis ended child birth deaths. Sallie Bernard got people to understand mercury was toxic. Relman foresaw and Angell witnessed a pharmaceutical takeover of medicine, Wakefield, like the others, has persevered in pursuit of modern day dangers inherent in vaccines. These individuals have all been subjected to ridicule. A whistleblower in the tobacco industry forced a Master Settlement Agreement.

# 18

Big Tobacco and King Pharma

Our vaccine situation today is in many respects comparable to a time period in the midst of our last century I witnessed as a child. I will recall those last fifty years for a reason, possibly linking then and now. I watched the health of my own tobacco smoking parents slowly deteriorate into fits of coughing, weight loss and profound shortness of breath. While our network media heavily subsidized by cigarette manufacturer's advertising dollars extolled the pleasures associated with smoking, the health of two generations was being riddled by ravages associated with tobacco. Our own family doctor, who smoked incessantly on three packs of Chesterfield cigarettes per day, would deny either his chest pains or my father's lung condition were due to their smoking habits.

Eventually a New York pulmonary specialist diagnosed my father's condition as emphysema, a rare form of terminal lung disease. With no proven treatments available, he recommended sand bags be placed on his stomach to help support his breathing. To his credit he also urged my father to stop smoking, because evidence was emerging there was a suspected link between smoking and a growing incidence of lung diseases, especially cancer. In 1962 a doctor warning a patient thinking about smoking would today be comparable to cautioning a patient an influenza vaccine could be harmful. Looking back media support combined with physician denial was a root cause for our failure to recognize what was and is happening around us. Parents and concerned doctors cannot afford to wait.

Smoking nightly news anchormen and doctors paraded out by Big tobacco denied any possible relationship between tobacco and cardio-respiratory diseases. These illnesses were just a coincidence. My father died of respiratory failure as I began my second year of medical school. On his death certificate a Yale University affiliated hospital pathologist wrote congestive heart failure. Intuitively, I knew it should have read death by tobacco in spite of our AMA's continuing claim smoking was safe.

By the time I graduated from medical school, a brave United States surgeon general was successful in getting a warning label placed on cigarette packages, although there would be no foreseeable AMA endorsement. Tobacco product sales did not decline, while the health of another generation did. Over ensuing years escalating epidemics of people dying from lung cancer and heart diseases continued as our tobacco controlled television network personnel refused to even acknowledge there might be evidence emerging of a link. Perhaps, time has now come for our current surgeon general to recommend a vaccine warning label indicating this product contains aluminum a proven neurotoxin dangerous to your health.

Our medical research community, conceivably in response to large grants of tobacco research money, generated study after study in support of tobacco's safety in spite of overwhelming evidence these papers were fraudulent and misleading. Of course, there were a few brave doctors bucking our established industry medical party line calling for a smoking ban until there was proof diseases of heart, lung and intestinal tracts were not being caused by tobacco smoking. People smoking by choice led to believe it was safe were becoming ill, being hospitalized and dying. Those realizing there was a danger tried to quit, but couldn't.

There was no doubt corruption existed at all levels of our tobacco industry, our medical community and our governmental regulatory agencies. Even with a warning label stating their product may be dangerous to health this industry had no problem distributing free sample packages to high school and college students as an acceptable way to add new users. P.T. Barnum, founder of the Greatest Show on

Earth, is believed to have said there is a sucker born every minute. It matters little whether Barnum or someone else actually provided us with this observation, the message rings true today as in yesteryear. How is it possible new physician generations can, once again, look at the evidence that our current epidemics parallel vaccine schedules and pretend not to see?

Big tobacco's success in getting their products into the mouths of our most vulnerable regardless of possible adverse events, without medical intervention, is a testimony to the truthfulness of Barnum's words. It would be fair to say, there were corporate executives and scientists in our tobacco industry with full knowledge of the danger who deliberately withheld critical information in their possession. Smokers without knowing or being warned about addiction were allowed to choose whether to smoke or not. Today, with vaccine mandates there is a correlation. An attempt is being made to deny infants, parents, caregivers and patients a similar right. Saying no, after being informed of possible risks, is an inalienable right.

Eventually, a tobacco inside whistleblower broke a silence on nicotine addiction in a New York Times story after being turned down by major networks, including 60 Minutes. Once again, editors at 60 Minutes had declined to do an important story about potential dire consequences for many, but not necessarily all smokers. Intellectually honest New York Times editors, perhaps understanding tobacco industry executives had deliberately withheld damaging information, approved this article for publication. The consequences would be far reaching. Addiction risk finally placed tobacco makers in an untenable position.

A state attorney general began to file suit against Big tobacco in an attempt to recoup his state's smoking related healthcare costs, especially for their medically indigent Medicaid and elderly Medicare insured victims. By 1998 tobacco's Big four agreed to a Master Settlement that would pay out over a quarter of a trillion dollars over twenty five years and billions of dollars annually forever, in order to remain in business. They knew their settlement costs would be fixed and recoverable by price increases as long as they were allowed to stay in business.

Some may consider this a brilliant one-sided tobacco industry legal victory. No doubt it was. Without worry about future product liability Big tobacco paid for a small percentage of total damages and stayed in business. In exchange for money, scientific medical fraud, industry and government corruption, future liability for deaths and disability were made to disappear forever. In essence, tobacco's slate was wiped clean. Addicted and those who would become addicted would be considered to have contributory negligence should they chose to continue or start smoking Many people passively exposed to tobacco smoke would continue to become ill. In some perverse way tobacco's Master Settlement Agreement money served societies greater good. Today our world's diversified tobacco industry is alive and well with major inroads into food, wine and vaccines. Something we allowed to happen and prosper, in spite of inflicting damages no one can calculate, got away from punishment. Meanwhile, approximately nine of every one hundred dollars in health insurance payments continue to go toward smoker medical costs.

Is it possible there will be similar insider stories emerging from our petrochemical and pharmaceutical industries concerning products having a similar potential to do more harm than actual benefit? Could these industries get away with using identical illegal, immoral, deceitful and unethical tactics? Vaccine makers with cunning legal help have already been given immunity thereby avoiding any possibility of a future vaccine damage related Master Settlement Agreement. Is it possible, if discovered, corporate, scientific and medical lies about product safety like their MMR or Round-Up could bring about their demise? Without informed doctors willing to speak up nothing will change. Pesticides, toxic metals, modified foods and harmful ingredients will be fed and injected without worry.

From all appearances vaccine insiders within our pharmaceutical industry have already planned out and executed their strategy by first obtaining gun point immunity from damages their products might be causing or be shown to cause. Clever structuring made taxpayers responsible for paying out all damages, if proven to be caused by vaccines. Adding a tax to each vaccine administered provided the funding necessary to compensate victims for death and disability. Vaccine makers likely knew there would be growing numbers of consequences associated with their infant and child cardio-respiratory, neurological and immune system tinkering. In order for vaccine makers to stay in business doctors would need to remain quiet and do what they were being told.

Manufactures smartly added another measure of safety for themselves by acknowledging and enumerating a sizable list of potential serious adverse events possibly associated with their individual vaccine products. Before 1986 vaccine makers may have suspected there would be a continuing epidemic of SIDS and a growing incidence of autism, asthma and autoimmune diseases that might someday become causally linked to their products. That day of reckoning could be delayed, if our VAERS was not allowed to accomplish injury documentation. Without sufficient submissions they could withstand subsequent cause-effect investigations. If there was only a very small percentage of adverse vaccine event reports coming in from millions upon millions of injections, there could be occasional settlements without alarms going off. If doctors and nurses were constantly being told vaccines were safe, rather than educated about VAERS, everything would be fine. Doctors could be paid to believe and cooperate.

Initially immunity from damages may have been reasonable in order to maintain vaccine production. However, in 1986 our vaccine schedule was limited to a few injections. No real safety studies existed. Nonetheless vaccine makers were being confronted by legitimate claims for damages. After obtaining immunity when problems with the mumps in their MMR and the cellular pertussis component of their DPT became associated with encephalitis, changes could be made to lessen infant risk without unfavorable publicity.

Although America's incidence of a child developing autism in 1980 was only one in five thousand, someone looking at a one in ten thousand incidence a decade before NCVIA should have seen something was going wrong. An unbridled escalation in autism numbers paralleling introductions of new vaccines flooding our infant market should have set off more alarms. With a growing number of post NCVIA vaccines, ACIP's childhood vaccine schedule would not be able to comfortably accommodate the total, unless multiple same day vaccines could be given. Our current dilemma created by multi-vaccine office visit decisions and verified by NICU studies has compounded our rapidly growing troubles. Just think, once again, about our incidence of autism in 1980 and 1990. Think about our medical excuses, such as, it was always there we are just becoming better at recognition. Or autism is an epidemic resulting from a genetic disease. Perhaps, autism results from a mother's inattention to her infant deserved attention. This Refrigerator mother theory's author was a fake doctor with no medical degree. Today our incidence is closer to one in thirty-six. Currently one in every fifty-nine children older than six years has autism. These unbelievable changes are not a coincidence they represent a consequence.

With growing quantities of aluminum being injected combined with continued use of mercury this situation should have been anticipated long before now. Studies showed aluminum and mercury toxicity existed well before vaccine immunity was granted. Legally vaccine makers knowing the adjuvant dangers should be held accountable for deliberate safety and efficacy deception prior to and following NCVIA, not unlike tobacco.

Our vaccine industry, in conjunction with doctors, have been allowed to go a step further by increasing numbers of first year vaccinations ten-fold over our past two decades. Adverse consequences during this same period were increasingly being recognized, but no one wanted or dared to connect the dots. There may be no vaccine maker protection under NCVIA or subsequent Supreme Court decisions if there have been lies about adjuvant safety accompanied by continued deceptive and false advertising. Is it possible removal of aluminum from vaccines would be equivalent to removing nicotine from cigarettes?

Never proven safety of single vaccines became same visit multi-injections consisting of combinations never previously tested for safety. Should we have at least expected numbers of adverse events would accelerate four or five-fold? Instead, once again, a well known pediatric expert irresponsibly proclaimed, babies could tolerate thousands of vaccines on the same day. When Dr. Offit made this proclamation there was evidence coming from ELBW infant NICU studies which confirmed monitored adverse cardio-respiratory events were being seen four times more frequently following administration of multi-vaccines. Is it possible this pediatric vaccine expert didn't read these studies, had no concern about these serious adverse events or the notion babies' lives matter?

Isn't it reasonable for expert researchers to extrapolate NICU findings to normal birth weight infants like Nicholas, Chris and Philip, who were not being monitored except by their mothers, following their DTP and TDaP injections? Isn't it reasonable for doctors, in general, to think twice before automatically giving an infant, who became ill on a prior occasion, another vaccine cocktail? Does anyone believe an infant sickened by vaccines at two or four months still deserves another round of similar shots at six months? If there are doctors still believing a moderate reaction to a bee sting or penicillin does not require future precautions, I suggest parents find doctors or mid-levels who know a lot more.

Dr. William Osler, considered the father of modern day medicine, once said never give two different medicines when one will suffice. He went on to say, if an adverse reaction occurs which one was responsible? Our committee responsible for our vaccine schedule and multi-vaccine recommendations without any consideration for serious known adverse events, a vulnerable infant population or reasonable genuinely frightened parents, will hopefully eventually come to a realization they have created more havoc, harm and suffering than imaginable for no conceivable or logical public good.

In *Dancing Cats Silent Canaries* I recommended parents refuse to give informed consent without reading vaccine manufacturer's package insert warnings about serious well documented adverse events including sudden death. Refusing to give consent is an exercise of a constitutional right. Everyone has a right to not smoke. All parents and caregivers must stand together and exercise similar rights regarding vaccinations. Freedom of choice must prevail over bullying doctors, nurses, judges, teachers and the media.

I recently read about a well known doctor who confessed he was a vaccine bully. Until he looked at his own practice and realized obvious vaccine consequences, he did not know better. He freely admitted children of vaccine refusers were his healthiest patients. Pediatricians seeing similar childhood vaccine damages insisting on parental vaccine compliance should be considered in breach of basic medical ethics.

Doctors with smoking and nonsmoking patients may have been able to draw similar conclusions. In the case of smoking, doctors were not being paid to encourage patient to increase their smoking.

A reasonable conclusion based upon my tobacco industry analogy is our vaccine industry can no longer be protected from product liability. Repeal of NCVIA should be a first step. Once repealed vaccine makers exposed to vaccine consequences will do one of two things either stop making vaccines or institute appropriate safety testing. Forcing vaccine makers to pay for past damages should result in a new vaccine Master Settlement Agreement designed to compensate victims of SIDS, autism, autoimmune diseases and neurological diseases of later years. Continued vaccinations, much like smoking, can no longer be defended or condoned. Vaccine makers must provide absolute proof adjuvants used in their products do not cause serious harm. Perhaps, before it is too late, they are already doing so by looking in a new direction.

Diversification has taken our tobacco industry into food, wines and health. Fate oftentimes takes unusual twists. Any suggestion tobacco and health would end up in one sentence might be considered laughable. A newly appointed head for our CDC suddenly resigned amid speculation she had invested heavily in tobacco. Casual observers might say it shouldn't be a big deal unless there was more to her story. Anyone knowing how close our CDC personnel are with vaccine makers had to be suspicious based upon prior incestuous relationships. A closer look revealed her speculation may have been kindled by the new direction tobacco was heading; namely, vaccines. Neither our tobacco nor vaccine industries would be looking at investing in agricultural based methodologies for creating vaccines unless there were good reasons. Cultivating vaccines in tobacco leaves must offer safety advantages over current methods. Wouldn't a merger of tobacco and vaccine maker interests be an ultimate irony? It might also be a sign something vaccine makers have been doing is terribly wrong. One comment might be cleaner safer vaccines through tobacco. If a safer genetically modified agricultural vaccine is in our future, can we simply ignore what has happened?

Is it possible with Glyphosate already being found in our current vaccines, will it not be found in tobacco leaves? Is it possible pharmaceutical companies working with tobacco and petrochemical companies will be able to produce cheaper, cleaner, safer, effective and more profitable vaccines with newer routes of administration without contaminating pesticides? Is it possible vaccine makers are preparing for a shift in the tide? I have a feeling vaccine makers are looking to cover their tracks with newer and safer vaccines before being caught.

# 19

## A Subtle Shift is Occurring

In apparent contradistinction to the past in June 2017 a top European Union (EU) court ruled vaccine makers under certain conditions can and should be held liable for damages. A vaccine could be considered defective, if there is specific and consistent evidence including the time between a vaccine's administration and onset of disease and similar reported cases in previously healthy individuals without a contributing family history. Although not widely reported, this is a quantum shift away from vaccine makers being held harmless. In other words a vaccine became a plausible explanation for a disease and consequently did not meet an implied and expected safety standard.

The EU ruling will in all likelihood evoke an equal and opposite response from our pharmaceutical vaccine industry and its medical and media allies. Vaccine package inserts already confess to dangers, including death and disability so how can reasonably intelligent people believe manufacturers deserve continued permanent freedom from liability based upon lies? Rather than wait manufacturers are rapidly attempting to implement plans to increase sales by force. In order to accomplish their financial objective mandatory regulations stripping parents and individuals of freedom of choice and informed consent are being enacted. Governments, legislators and doctors perhaps, already corrupted by prior gifts are voting for statutory mandates alleging our public good is being threatened by growing numbers of pro-choice informed skeptics, rather than by our existing pandemic.

Instead of agreeing to common sense logic for enacting the *Precautionary Principle* followed by a well controlled study comparing the health of vaccinated and unvaccinated groups our vaccine industry with the full support of the AMA and AAP want no further evidence which might threaten profits and add to parental fears. Inherent fears such a study might create a worst case scenario within vaccinated groups is being echoed in words from our 2003 IOM, no more science is necessary the case in favor of vaccine safety is closed.

Any outcome from a prospective or retroactive study will not be of benefit to either vaccine makers or traditional medical doctors. It would prove vaccines are neither safe nor very effective. Although safety lack is already well known a lack of effectiveness has become evident with outbreaks of measles, mumps and whooping cough, mainly in vaccinated groups, rather than the unvaccinated. To make matters worse for manufacturers within their own companies and our CDC there are scientists who have already admitted to fraud. Rather than continue to hide their damaging testimony agreeing to a major schedule delay might slow current epidemics without any high level admission there is a real and present danger.

Without a study proving vaccines are safe combined with growing hesitancy and outright resistance, vaccine makers are shifting in response to their apparent vulnerability. Turning to legislators to enact laws with penalties for parental non-compliance is nothing more than an act of desperation. Increasing numbers of compensation awards will have no immediate impact on profitability, but in order to continue their growth mandates will be necessary. Mandates will not work. Protesters with help from doctors, nurses, medical exemptions and home schooling will simply find a path around any new obstacles. No matter what mandates cannot replace proofs for safety.

A look at history will reveal other frightening truths that demonstrate manufacturers come first and human beings last. Asbestos, a deadly fiber proven responsible for countless Mesothelioma deaths has not been banned in the United States. It is now present everywhere in our environment. Workers demolishing older apartment, office and school buildings are required by law to wear protective masks and clothing with annual respiratory exams. In the 1930's a doctor who proclaimed asbestos was killing workers was threatened with the loss of his medical license if he persisted warning those being exposed. Does this sound familiar? A doctor prohibited from practicing by Maryland's medical board for pointing a finger at vaccines being a likely cause for his son's autism has been awarded damages. This signals another shift is occurring because board members who voted to revoke his license have been ruled personally liable for damages. Is it possible school board members invoking mandates will need to be prepared for similar?

Eventually in the case of asbestos modern day evidence became insurmountable. Rather than try to ban this harmful product it is simpler to pay damages. Sadly, since dedicating my 2010 book to my younger brother, a Mesothelioma victim, he succumbed three years later. Although his incredible will to live took him to congressional offices attempting to help others, he was told not to be hopeful, a Supreme Court Justice had once been an asbestos industry defense attorney. There have been other poisonings, perhaps deliberate where warnings were calculatingly withheld, at least until the resultant crisis became too overwhelming to ignore, as in our current Flint, Michigan and widespread opioid crisis.

Epidemic opioid use and related deaths has been ongoing and growing thanks in large part to manufacturing freedom, weak legislative regulations, liberal well paid physician prescribing and a growing demand oftentimes encouraged by affordable medical insurance plans. In addition to narcotic makers, doctors, health care facilities and entrepreneurs have capitalized handsomely on a vulnerable and now addicted population subset. Taxpayers are ultimately paying for the consequences. Perhaps, there will be a shift toward safer physician prescribing patterns when it comes to opiates and vaccines rather than continued talk.

A few years ago while fulfilling my continuing education requirements, I took an online continuing medical education course that extolled major quality of life benefits of opioids. This course was possibly funded by the industry and endorsed by the medical licensing board in a state that was being supportive of a burgeoning number of for profit pain management centers. Once local media climbed aboard it was only a matter of time before there would be an unprecedented shift in what was considered an opioid greater good. Favorable legislation made production and distribution of opiate drugs possible. The pharmaceutical industry flourished with the creation of addiction treatment centers. Our pharmaceutical industry simply shifted by increasing rather than decreasing costs for their lifesaving treatment products. Gradually answers to my continuing medical education questions about quality of life with opiate prescribing once again changed with closures of for profit pain centers. Audaciously our vaccine industry is attempting a shift to mandates forcing healthcare workers to comply with prescribing their dangerous vaccine products. More doctors saying no to prescribing and administering vaccines will be a worthy but unacceptable shift.

Personal freedom of choice legislation in Texas recently dealt well paid legislators and pharmaceutical lobbyists an unexpected resounding defeat, while other financially motivated doctors and legislators in other states attempt to follow California's SB277 lead as parental resistance mounts. The shift taking place against vaccine and law maker collusion is becoming obvious. California's Richard Pan is both a state senator and a pediatrician. SB277 can be attributed to Pan and the reported contributions he and his senate colleagues received from vaccine lobbyists. The existing corruption between doctors, the vaccine industry and government is personified by this man. His next objective is to censor social media postings he does not believe are appropriate. No one with intact moral integrity and intellectual honesty can afford to stand on the sidelines and watch people like Pan promote a continued decline in our children's health and First Amendment rights in America. An immediate shift to getting rid of congressmen and state legislators who take pharmaceutical and petrochemical money in return for attempting to strip Americans of their rights is our best immediate course.

The subtle shift in liability that is occurring will grow with the realization we can no longer trust in our current system or our elected officials. We are being forced to resort to our legal profession to protect our rights. Those parents and caregivers who choose to refuse to consent to avoidable and unsafe vaccines and the awakened doctors willing to listen and provide possible lifesaving medical exemptions will need help. The probable liability associated with IRB and medical board member decisions will become more apparent as information of the hidden vaccination dangers are exposed. Doctors attempting to discharge children of pro-choice parents from their practices should be formally reported to their state's medical society and licensing board. If a doctor refuses to complete a VAERS form or medical exemption parents believe is justifiable a complaint to the state licensing board may also become appropriate.

# 20

## Is this the Brave New World?

Fifty years after receiving my George Washington University medical degree, serving as a doctor with our Navy during Vietnam and helping to create emergency medicine as a new specialty, I find it necessary to continue speaking out. Frankly, I am both ashamed and frightened. There is already enough evidence to conclude our toxic environment is taking an incredible human toll in terms of lives, neurological and autoimmune disorders. Our age of better living through chemicals began in earnest during our last century with introductions of PVC products to a growing list of chemical herbicides and pesticides. A brief victory with a ban on DDT did not stop newer more treacherous products, such as Glyphosate and genetically modified foods (GMO's), from reaching markets without need for safety testing.

Lead, a major component of gasoline, paints and some cosmetics became recognized as a neurotoxic substance, but its removal did not take this heavy metal out of older paint, soil or already contaminated water supplies. Arsenic, heavily used in mining and fungicides, mercury, used in over the counter medicines and dental amalgams, joined cadmium, chromium, and nickel in our public water supplies and food chains. Coal burning clouds dumped methyl mercury into our oceans and aquatic foods to the point tuna fish was not recommended for consumption, especially for those pregnant. Tobacco use, proclaimed medically safe, intensified with favorable media publicity adding to an array of toxic poisons already adversely affecting human cardio-respiratory, immune and neurological systems.

Industries promoting better chemicals and safe tobacco were joined by the pharmaceutical and fast food industry in an all out assault on the human condition in an emerging brave new world. Drugs for a myriad of newly discovered psychological, gastrointestinal, cardio-respiratory, hematologic and immune disease diagnoses rapidly multiplied in spite of their likely potential for causing physical dependency, rebound and serious adverse events. With cause effect correlations products were removed and victim damages were paid. Without discovery bad events were soon outweighing good, but business went on as usual.

Chemical, tobacco and pharmaceutical industry sales representative fanned out to inform law makers, farmers, smokers-to-be and our medical profession everything was good. Doctor cooperation was enhanced with impressive multi-level perks. Frank kickbacks couched in politer terms soon became abundant. Doctors were wined and dined into submission. Slowly with declining pharmaceutical sales, growing suspicions about safety and potential litigation the giants had to adapt. Rather than simply deny poisonous chemical products that were openly illegally being dumped with safe passage into public water supplies and vulnerable children and pay for the cleanup, the doors began to close. Clean ups became an obligation for taxpayers. Larger companies expanded their legal departments, sponsored contradictory medical science, added highly paid lobbyists, gained positive media coverage with advertising and began campaign funding for favorite trustworthy candidates for higher offices. Our pharmaceutical industry took a giant step toward diversification by creating newer vaccines for societies greater good. The vaccine industry grew based upon the premise and promise childhood illnesses could safely and effectively become a thing of our past. Unfortunately, vaccine damages quickly became apparent necessitating corrective action. Vaccines soon became toxic tipping points for many children in our brave new world.

Dismayed by successful lawsuits vaccine makers needed a new world order without liability risk. They got what they wanted and paid for. Without need to show mercury or aluminum could be safely injected into infants and children, a new race was on. Proofs either for efficacy or safety would not be necessary. Vaccines, dubbed our biggest advance in childhood medicine, would be sold by doctors, especially pediatricians, and a vaccine schedule endorsed by our CDC, ACIP and AAP. Their strategy following NCVIA would only be successful, if doctors did not understand the requirements of VAERS. Minimizing adverse event reports would guarantee unlimited growth in sales of existing vaccine products and those to come.

Looking back I cannot state with absolute certainty there was a direct effort made to educate doctors about the importance of their roles in being suspicious any death or illness following a vaccination might represent an adverse event. After intense questioning, I am certain ACEP never received direct notification about emergency physician responsibilities. More concerning to me is the fact that I am unaware of any communication between CDC, DHHS, vaccine makers and ACEP leadership or more than 25,000 physician members concerning our vaccine adverse warning responsibilities. Consequently, there has been no formal ACEP organizational reporting policy or any significant educational programs designed to inform emergency physicians what they should be looking for in order to abide by the law and initiate reports. As a consequence, NCVIA has been our vaccine makers Trojan horse. Their camouflaged gift to medicine must be eliminated. Any good intended by this act was deliberately vacated by a failure to communicate physician responsibilities. Deliberately failing to include emergency physicians in their safety net and adding physician compliance payments compounded our vaccine industry's intended deception.

I believe educating doctors, especially those manning more than five thousand emergency facilities, about VAERS with the establishment of an EMR would have provided concurrent submissions ultimately showing the seriousness of what appears to be the major role vaccines are playing in newer childhood diseases seldom seen 50 years ago. I believe within one year emergency department adverse event submissions alone would have demanded invocation of a vaccine *Precautionary Principle* and lead to the repeal of NCVIA. Instead any promises of safety were systematically overcome by product promotional propaganda emphasizing only what could be construed as positive benefits.

Shielding doctors and parents from a growing vaccine downside would be manageable with fake science, controlled media and money.

Toxicity, especially for our young, caused by chemicals, mercury aluminum combinations still in vaccines, rampant medical denial and emerging evidence showing vaccines have created a problem for our new not so brave world can no longer be disregarded. What has transpired should be construed as criminal intent. Education will lead to the evidence which has been deliberately allowed to go missing. This evidence will show once and for all we have not been given correct answers. Any safety promises given have been broken again and again. Physicians have purposely been misguided. Those able to see what is happening are being threatened. Doctors are being torn apart by fear. Fear of losing vaccination income is compounded by a fear they are witnessing the reasons why their practices have dramatically been changing with more unhealthy patients than ever imaginable. Many are so frightened they refuse to even talk about vaccine injuries. They become angry at the very word. Many don't want to consider any possibility they have participated in our detrimental vaccine age. Most still refuse to consider even a remote possibility something they did do or did not do has been a major contributing factor.

Trying to process a new reality is far too difficult for most physicians. Better to believe vaccines have always been and will remain safe provides a relative comfort zone. Fortunately, doctors are slowly beginning to see and are refusing to do what they are being told. Eventually, there will be a fuller realization they are no longer working for patients or themselves but rather insurance, pharmaceutical and healthcare corporation demands. Our growing suicide rate among physicians may ultimately be traced to productivity demands associated with poorer outcomes and recognition there is no way injected poisons can do no harm. I can no longer see a role for our current obsolete and dangerous vaccine program and continued physician payments in a braver physician world. Stopping this man-made plague sooner rather than later is possible. Doctors must decide it is time to get off the CDC, HHS, ACIP and AAP powered vaccine merry-go-round now spinning out of control.

Recently after speaking with the new ACEP leadership about VAERS and a need for physician education, it dawned on me that most of what is missing may already be in insurance company or third party hands. Placing further demands on stressed out emergency physicians seemed simple, but might also be too much to ask. Even if there was a thousand fold first year increase in VAERS submissions, there would be no guarantee something good might happen. Reports suddenly coming from our nation's emergency departments, showing how serious our vaccine dilemma is could flagrantly be ignored by resistant doctors, agencies, legislators and manufacturers. It would also be unlikely our other medical organizations would be supportive. Simply put, when it comes to vaccines, everyone, except parents and their babies, have too much to lose. Regardless of outcome, I realized help would still be needed from my emergency colleagues, while I directed my attention to our insurance industry. Hopefully, a resolution will be introduced and approved at ACEP's 50th Anniversary Scientific Assembly in San Diego, California in 2018.

Meanwhile getting to existing information under ordinary circumstances should not be too difficult, provided of course, there is nothing being hidden and there is nothing to hide. Dates of office visits for vaccinations and subsequent visits to the same office, an urgent care or ED for an illness or unexpected death within 30 days should already be available or easily searched for within HIPPA guidelines. If there is damaging evidence in insurance company records, the failure to report serious adverse vaccine events might actually have been an executive decision. Although vaccine injury law allows third party submissions, perhaps as long as no one asks, it could be construed as an accidental oversight. The far more haunting thought is it has been a deliberate cover-up.

Looking at our current situation I cannot help but feel fearful. With NICU studies miserably failing to confirm vaccine safety, rising autism rates, unexplained infant deaths, mandates with penalties and insurance information being withheld, possibly there is no one in meaningful authority who might want to know why this has happened. Although there might be enough evidence in insurance company and other third party files, unless a brave state attorney general decided to take action by asking for cooperation our status quo would likely continue. If only Mississippi's state attorney general decided to ask his state's Medicaid program to provide never reported data, it might be a gigantic first step in the right direction. There has to be a reason for this state's poor childhood health and high infant death rate. A mandatory vaccine policy combined with Medicaid payment data and childhood illness diagnostic codes might provide a correlation with death rates and disease. If nothing else there may be enough evidence to stop Mississippi's mandate and restore informed consent, medical exemptions, First Amendment and Civil rights.

Analyzing this state's Medicaid database would be a huge but extremely worthwhile gamble. On the one hand, our CDC, vaccine industry and Supreme Court could be vindicated for past decisions and everyone could move forward based upon an absence of significant temporal evidence of vaccination harm. Vindication followed by cooperation would be a huge victory for the status quo. Finding temporal evidence might represent a huge victory for vaccine safety doubters and possibly uncover a group of unrecognized victims. Either way, this could be a new beginning or a concluding chapter, for our current vaccine industry. Without going into detail I believe our CDC, by supporting a transparent and honest in depth look at Mississippi's children, could become the biggest winner.

Having stated what needs to be said, there is probably no one mothers can currently trust other than their maternal instinct. Parents must invoke their own *Precautionary Principle* before it's too late. In the meantime I intend to ask for help from insurance claim processors to whistle-blow important data in order to answer reasonable questions about vaccine dates followed by death or illness in accordance with current law. I believe this industry also has retrospective information about the current health of both vaccinated and unvaccinated children. I cannot imagine opposition to insurance company VAERS information coming from the AAP, practicing physicians or Dr. Paul Offit. In the aftermath our brave new world may be forced to deal with a return of some childhood illnesses, if insurance data shows chickenpox is less deadly than injected aluminum.

It is doubtful, either our government or medical profession will realize what has been happening until more doctors join with protesters who have chosen to stand up and attempt to be heard above bottom line serving proclamation noise. I know what I have seen and now feel more compelled than ever to determine the reasons. Few can understand my enthusiasm lining up for Salk's polio vaccine. It was my ultimate joy not knowing there would be future risk for polio from newer vaccines. If I had known my promised protection might be responsible for future vaccine maker immunity, I may have said no thank you. Immunity from liability was never earned by an industry parents are being asked to trust.

The time has come to call an industry on its callous disregard for babies' lives and safety in the name of money. It is time for our congressmen to take an informed look at the carnage created by NCVIA and paid for Supreme Court decisions, devastating vaccine mandates and cruel almost inhumane, criminal NICU studies injecting aluminum into ELBW infants, children and teenage boys and girls. It is also time to stop medical experts from abusing and bullying informed and uninformed parents and caregivers about an absolute need to have their infants and children injected with vaccines unavoidably unsafe in the face of a worldwide pandemic likely attributable to these same unsafe products.

I implore my medical colleagues, esteemed members of our legal profession and state legislators to say no to vaccine money and mandates. The legal scale balance has been blindly shifting into a danger, far in excess of safety zone, demanding a vaccine moratorium for the sake of newborns, infants and children. Our attempt in the name of childhood illnesses prevention has become an overall dismal medical failure, unless available evidence is allowed to become known proving babies are not dying or suffering serious adverse events within thirty days of their vaccinations. If evidence shows our vaccine adverse reporting system could have stopped our current epidemics we, as physicians, have allowed this to happen by not paying attention and turning our backs on the facts and our patients. Physicians may not have another opportunity to take back what has been lost The practice of do no harm medicine is in extreme jeopardy.

It has been reported things may be worsening. I have clearly stated my medical opinion about Gardasil. Sales of HPV vaccines with increasing strains and similar amounts of aluminum are not meeting fiscal forecasts. Due to a lower than expected uptake, I recently became aware Merck may be planning on a University of Alabama (UAB) maternity ward vaccine promotion. Merck proposes giving Gardasil injections to 16-26 year old girls hospitalized following labor and delivery. Although I am uncertain whether this is true, there should be some significant concern regarding both Merck and UAB's hospital board of directors assuming this is not a planned study needing an IRB approval. If board members agree to allow Merck's Gardasil, even with patient informed consent, they may be placing themselves at personal risk. Doctors and nurses, who fail to disclose proposed vaccine benefits with risks associated with aluminum injections, will likely find themselves also at legal risk. Insurance companies paying for these injections or for physician performance may also become liable.

Hopefully this is strictly an attempt to sell vaccines not a study. No civilized IRB, no matter how much vaccine money has been promised, should even consider approving this do or die experiment. No new mother should agree to be given either a free or insurance covered injection without consulting with an attorney. No studies have been done showing this vaccine's possible adverse effects on fertility. Gardasil injections on maternity wards should never be allowed without entering each recipient into a comprehensive study protocol with long-term follow up extending to their babies. What will happen to mothers on UAB's maternity wards that refuse? Will journalists and comedians want punishments? What will happen to doctors or nurses who decline to participate in this planned atrocious practice? What will happen to babies of nursing mothers when hep B injected aluminum and other chemicals join together in newborn brains? There will be consequences, if only a minority of mothers develop serious adverse events.

In conclusion, parents, caregivers, physicians, physician assistants, nurse practitioners, nurses and medical assistants must understand vaccines have never been proven safe. Trusting our vaccine industry is no longer possible. Trusting doctors who believe vaccines are safe is a mistake. Allowing vaccine mandates will become a monumental freedom of choice travesty. Re-electing pro-chemical and pro-vaccine people to our state and federal legislative offices will quicken our demise. Restoring vaccine maker liability for adverse event damages is a necessity. Adding legal discovery to our vaccine injury compensation process is essential. Every possible vaccine related death or long term injury over the past ten years must be uncovered and reported from whatever source in possession of the medical information. Turning back our vaccine maker's timetable by invoking a precautionary ban on vaccines and their toxic adjuvants until reliable transparent data can be gathered and viewed is an acceptable option, if repeal of NCVIA is not forthcoming. Parents in increasing numbers refusing vaccines combined with physicians approving medical exemptions for reasons mentioned will help create order out of vaccine chaos.

*Children are the World's most valuable resource and its best hope for the future. John F. Kennedy*

*Vaccination is barbarous practice and one of the most fatal of all the delusion current in our time. Conscientious objectors to vaccinations should stand alone, if need be, against the whole world in defense of their conviction*
*Mahatma Gandhi*

*Never do anything against conscience even if the state demands it,*
*Albert Einstein*

Printed in the United States
By Bookmasters